Pharmacology

Self-assessment Questions for Students

Second Edition

Rosemarie Einstein

BSc(Hons), PhD
Department of Pharmacology, University of Sydney

Butterworths

Sydney—London—Boston—Singapore
Toronto—Wellington
1989

National Library of Australia
Cataloguing-in-Publication entry

Pharmacology, self-assessment questions for students.

2nd ed.
Includes index.
ISBN 0 409 30127 2.

1. Pharmacology — Examinations, questions, etc. I.
Einstein, Rosemarie.

615.1076

Printed in Australia by The Book Printer.

CONTRIBUTORS
University of Sydney, Department of Pharmacology

R D Allan, BSc, PhD, Senior Lecturer
S Armsworth, BSc, Dip Ed, M Med Sci, Tutor
A Cincotta, BPharm, Dip Hosp Pharm, Tutor
R Einstein, BSc, PhD, Senior Lecturer
D M Jackson, BPharm, MSc, PhD, Associate Professor
G A R Johnston, BSc, MSc, PhD, FRACI, Professor
E J Mylecharane, BPharm, PhD, Senior Lecturer
J P Seale, MB BS, PhD, FRACP, Associate Professor
J Shaw, MB BS, PhD, FRACP, Professor of Clinical Pharmacology
I Spence, BSc, PhD, Lecturer
G A Starmer, BPharm, MSc, PhD, Associate Professor
D M Temple, BSc, MSc, PhD, Associate Professor
S D Whicker, BSc, Tutor.

Research Associates and guest lecturers in the Department provided some of the questions in this book. We are grateful for their contribution to the teaching and assessment of our students.

CONTENTS

PREFACE

Our Department of Pharmacology has been using objective examinations for students in Medicine, Pharmacy, Science and Veterinary Science for the past eleven years. These objective examinations, short answer questions, assignments and practical classes all contribute to the students' assessment. The shortcomings of this type of examination are appreciated but the lack of alternative methods which provide rapid assessment of up to 1000 students at any one time leaves us no choice but to continue using objective question examinations. The student answer sheets are computer-marked at the Tertiary Education Research Unit, University of New South Wales. The computer output provides information relating to the examination performance of the students, the percentage of students answering each question correctly and the coefficient of discrimination for each question. The latter gives some indication of the ability of the question to discriminate between the good and poor students.

We store a bank of 5000 questions on computer. Constant review of the bank includes adding the information relating to student performance for each question each time it is set, deleting questions which have become outdated or which are found to be ambiguous, misleading or otherwise unsatisfactory and adding new questions.

The questions in this book have been selected from the bank and therefore reflect the content of the lectures for our undergraduate courses in all faculties. Some of the questions are suitable only for students from particular faculties and some apply only to New South Wales or Australia. There is, however, a large number of questions with which all students may assess their progress. Every effort has been made to avoid duplication of subject matter, to ensure that the questions are not ambiguous and to provide accurate answers. We would welcome comments relating to these issues from all those using the book.

Using this book

The book cannot replace study. It is primarily intended to be used some time after a period of study, to test understanding and retention of learned material. I suggest you do not attempt to answer questions on a topic immediately after you have studied it because this may only assess short term memory function. Answering questions correctly a few days after the study period is a more reliable indication that you have understood and retained the information.

The answers to questions can be found at the end of each chapter. We have consciously decided against including explanations of the answers. It is your responsibility to consult your textbooks, lecture notes or teachers for explanations. The search for this information is a form of active study and plays a major role in the learning and reinforcing process. If you have answered a question incorrectly and simply check the correct answer in the list at the end of the chapter, it is unlikely that you will remember it. You will benefit far more if you spend some time checking the information in your notes and textbooks. Actively dealing with the subject matter will help your learning of the subject most effectively.

Questions for self-testing may be chosen either by working through an appropriate chapter or by reference to the keyword index at the end of the book. The index has been compiled from keywords as they appear in the questions, i.e. names of individual drugs or drug groups, naturally-occurring active substances (hormones, neurotransmitters, autacoids, etc.) and disease states. Those questions marked with a "V" have been set primarily for students of Veterinary Science and are not applicable for students in other faculties.

The questions in this book are of five different types. In increasing order of complexity these are:

TYPE 1 - **TRUE / FALSE**
Each question consists of a statement. Indicate whether it is true or false.

TYPE 2 - **CORRECT OPTION**
Each question consists of a stem and up to five options or five sentences, only one of which is correct. Indicate the correct option.

TYPE 3 - **INCORRECT OPTION**
The same as Type 2, except the single incorrect option should be indicated.

TYPE 4 - **MULTIPLE CHOICE QUESTION (MCQ)**
Each question consists of a stem and up to 5 options or five sentences, a number of which are correct.
Answer: A if only (i), (ii) and (iii) are correct
         B if only (i) and (iii) are correct
         C if only (ii) and (iv) are correct
         D if only (iv) is correct
         E if all are correct.

TYPE 5 - **ASSERTION / REASON**
Each question consists of an assertion and a reason.
Answer: A if the assertion and the reason are true statements and the reason is the correct explanation of the assertion
         B if the assertion and the reason are true statements but the reason is not a correct explanation of the assertion
         C if the assertion is true, but the reason is a false statement
         D if the assertion is false, but the reason is a true statement
         E if both the assertion and reason are false statements.

Good luck with your studying!

September, 1989   *Rosemarie Einstein*

1 Introduction

TRUE / FALSE

1.1   Tachyphylaxis is a form of resistance to the action of a drug.

1.2   The content of pharmacologically active alkaloids in a species of plant may vary between individual plants.

1.3   Drugs with different mechanisms of action may achieve the same effect.

1.4   Side effects of drugs are not always adverse.

1.5   All useful drugs have a clearly defined mechanism of action.

1.6   All registered drugs have a generic or non-proprietary name.

1.7   The chemical name for a drug is rarely the same as the non-proprietary name.

1.8   A single drug may have many trade names.

1.9   Receptors for drug action may exhibit stereospecificity.

1.10 Receptors may be "down-regulated" by removal of endogenous inhibitors.

1.11 Multiple binding sites may interact in a co-operative manner to influence dose-response relationships.

1.12 Negative co-operativity results in very steep dose-response relationships.

1.13 The dissociation constant of a drug is independent of the lifetime of the drug-receptor complex.

1.14 Scatchard plots are used to determine the rate of drug action.

1.15 A curvilinear Scatchard plot indicates that a drug may exhibit co-operativity or bind to more than one site.

1.16 Ligand binding studies are essential for the development of new drugs.

1.17 Radioligand binding experiments usually cannot be used to distinguish between agonists and antagonists.

1.18 A graph of the effect of a drug plotted against the logarithm of its dose is usually sigmoid in shape.

1.19   The quantal dose-response relationship provides a measure of the variation in doses needed to produce an all-or-none effect in a group of subjects.

1.20   A response does not necessarily follow the interaction of a drug with a binding site on a cell.

1.21   The negative logarithm of the molar concentration of an agonist drug, corresponding to the centre of symmetry of a log-dose response curve, is a measure of the potency of the agonist for the receptor.

1.22   The binding affinity of a drug is directly related to its efficacy of action.

1.23   The affinity of a drug for a receptor can be measured for both agonists and antagonists.

1.24   Agonist drugs which act on the same receptors have parallel log-dose response curves.

1.25   When the potencies of two drugs are compared, the more potent has the greater EC_{50} value.

1.26   When conventional log dose-response curves are plotted to compare the results of LD_{50} determinations of two substances, the curve for the more toxic chemical will be on the right hand side.

1.27   Antagonist drugs are molecules which have affinity for the receptor but do not have the ability to stimulate the receptor.

1.28   Antagonist drugs have high intrinsic activity.

1.29   A drug which is described as a partial agonist can act as an antagonist.

1.30   Functional antagonism occurs when two agonist drugs, interacting through two independent receptor systems, cause effects which counteract each other.

1.31   Non-specific antagonism occurs when the affinity of an antagonist for its receptor increases as the dose is raised.

1.32   The pA_2 value for atropine at a muscarinic receptor should be the same whether acetylcholine or muscarine is used as the agonist.

1.33-1.36
        Drug W is a full agonist
        Drug X is a competitive antagonist of drug
        Drug Y is a functional antagonist of drug
        Drug Z is a non-competitive antagonist of drug

1.33   Drug Y interacts with a receptor system distinct from the receptor system of drug W.

1.34   The maximal effect obtained with drug W would decrease in the presence of increasing concentrations of drug X.

1.35   In the presence of drug Z, the slope of the dose-response curve to drug W would show a parallel shift to the right.

1.36   The maximum effect obtainable with drug W would decrease in the presence of increasing concentrations of drug Z.

1.37   Inhaled drugs enter the body very slowly.

1.38   Following oral administration to man, drugs are absorbed primarily in the intestine.

1.39   Following the administration of a single oral dose of a drug, peak concentrations in the plasma usually occur between 1 and 3 hours.

1.40   The rate of absorption of an acidic drug from the stomach is enhanced by the co-administration of sodium bicarbonate.

1.41   Use of a depot preparation results in slow absorption.

1.42   Administration of a drug as a depot salt is the only effective method of increasing its half-life.

1.43   Absorption of drugs through mucous membranes is more effective than through skin.

1.44   After subcutaneous injection most drug molecules are taken up mainly by the lymphatic capillaries.

The rate of absorption of drugs through the intestinal wall:

1.45   varies directly with the area of absorption surface.

1.46   always depends on a positive concentration gradient between intestinal contents and plasma.

1.47   The distribution of thiopentone in the body is initially controlled by fat deposits.

1.48   Dangerous drug interactions may occur if one drug displaces another from protein binding sites.

1.49   Active transport mechanisms are responsible for most aspects of drug distribution in the body.

1.50   Binding of a drug to plasma proteins aids its transport into the central nervous system.

1.51   Plasma protein binding of drugs may serve as the means of transport of some drugs in the body.

1.52   Lipid solubility is the most important factor in influencing drug entry into the brain.

1.53   Acidic drugs tend not to be reabsorbed from the renal tubule.

1.54   A lipophilic drug, after i.v. administration, accumulates slowly in the brain.

1.55   Prodrugs are designed to undergo metabolism to inactive metabolites that are readily excreted.

1.56   Drugs must be metabolised before they are excreted.

1.57   Oxidation of drugs *in vivo* is usually carried out by hepatic microsomal enzymes.

1.58   Most drugs must be conjugated before they can be metabolised in the liver.

1.59   The more water-soluble a drug, the longer is its duration of action.

1.60   In progressive liver disease, phase 2 biotransformations are impaired whilst phase 1 biotransformations are preserved.

1.61   Monoamine oxidase A is found in the liver and gastrointestinal tract.

1.62   Deprenyl is a selective inhibitor for monoamine oxidase type A.

Drug biotransformation:

1.63   occurs predominantly in the liver.

1.64   usually converts polar molecules to non-polar molecules.

1.65   may be responsible for the mutagenicity of certain drugs.

1.66   is responsible for the hepatotoxicity of paracetamol.

1.67   always utilises energy from ATP.

1.68   usually increases the drug's water solubility.

1.69   The rate of urinary excretion of a strongly basic drug is enhanced by the co-administration of ammonium chloride.

1.70   The excretion of a weakly acidic drug may be decreased by decreasing urinary pH with ammonium chloride.

1.71   Drugs with a high affinity for circulating protein have a high rate of urinary excretion.

1.72   Drug excretion into bile may result in its reabsorption.

1.73   Species variations in responses to a given drug may result from different pharmacokinetic patterns.

1.74   Zero-order kinetics apply when the rate of absorption is a function of the amount of drug available for absorption.

1.75   Zero-order kinetics apply if the elimination of a drug involves a saturable rate-limiting process.

1.76   The rate constant of elimination of a drug is equal to the sum of the rate constants of biotransformation and excretion.

1.77   When drugs are administered orally, the larger the dose the more rapidly the maximum plasma level is obtained.

1.78   The loading dose of a drug is the product of the desired plasma concentration and the clearance of the drug.

1.79   The volume of distribution of a drug is equal to the total amount of drug in the body divided by the concentration of drug in the plasma.

1.80   The volume of distribution of a drug cannot exceed the volume of total body water.

1.81   The volume of distribution of a drug can only exceed the volume of total body water for highly lipid-soluble drugs.

1.82   When a drug is extensively bound to extra-vascular binding sites, its apparent volume of distribution may be much greater than the total body water.

1.83   The area under the plasma concentration-time curve is a function of dose, volume of distribution and the rate of elimination.

1.84   The fraction of an oral dose absorbed can be calculated if the areas under the plasma drug concentration vs time curves for oral and intravenous doses are known.

1.85   In the equation to determine the plasma concentration of a drug at time t after i.v. administration, the number of exponential factors in the equation is equal to the number of compartments into which the drug is distributed.

1.86   Dose-dependent kinetics describe the behaviour of a drug in a one-compartment model.

1.87   A one-compartment pharmacokinetic model is a valid approximation, only if distribution from the central compartment to one or more peripheral compartments reaches equilibrium slowly.

1.88   The half-life of a drug is the time from administration until its maximum effect is reduced by half.

1.89   The biological half-life of a drug is usually less than the plasma half-life.

1.90   The effect of a drug may still be evident long after all the drug has been excreted.

1.91   If a drug has a biological half-life of 6 hours, all its effects will have worn off after 24 hours.

1.92   If the clearances of drug A and drug B are the same but the distribution volume of drug A is greater than the distribution volume of drug B, then the half-life of elimination for drug A will be less than that for drug B.

1.93   Drugs which are highly lipid-soluble are unlikely to give rise to problems of cumulative toxicity.

1.94   If the "first-pass" metabolism of a drug is extensive it will be necessary to prescribe a smaller oral dose to patients with liver disease.

1.95   The pharmacological effect of a drug is always proportional to its plasma concentration.

1.96   For most drugs there is a well-defined range of plasma concentrations within which their therapeutic effects will occur.

If the plasma concentration of a drug is plotted against the time following the administration of a single oral dose:

1.97   the area under the curve will be independent of the rate of absorption.

1.98   a symmetrical bell-shaped curve would indicate that metabolism by the liver is important in the disposal of the drug.

1.99   the elimination "half-life" of the plasma concentration could be calculated from the time taken to reach peak concentration.

1.100 the peak concentration will depend only on the rate and extent of absorption of the drug from the gastrointestinal tract.

After i.v. administration of a drug, pharmacokinetic data which fit a single compartment model can be used to calculate:

1.101 the absorption rate constant for the drug.

1.102 the volume of distribution.

1.103 the half-life of the drug.

1.104 the extent of absorption of the drug after oral administration.

If a patient is receiving a drug by continuous intravenous infusion:

1.105   increasing the rate of infusion reduces the time required to achieve a steady-state plasma level.

1.106   decreasing the rate of infusion decreases the steady-state plasma level.

1.107   Bioavailability is expressed as the percentage of a given dose of drug which appears in the systemic circulation.

1.108   The bioavailability of a drug is directly proportional to its first-pass metabolism in the liver.

1.109   Clinical problems may arise from the variable bioavailability of warfarin.

1.110   Two tablets of digoxin made by different manufacturers will always have the same bioavailability provided the dosage forms each contain 100mg of the pure drug.

1.111   Problems of bioavailability are most likely to arise with drugs which are poorly water-soluble.

1.112   The bioavailability of a drug is controlled in part by its lipid/water partition coefficient.

1.113   Drugs which are rapidly absorbed into body fat always have a short duration of action.

1.114   The more water-soluble a drug, the longer is its duration of action.

CORRECT OPTION

1.115   The development of tolerance describes a situation where:
A.   the dose of a drug must be increased to maintain a given effect
B.   a response of unusually large magnitude is produced by a normal dose
C.   a patient experiences withdrawal symptoms if the drug is not given at regular intervals
D.   an unusual type of response is produced by a drug
E.   the patient is unable to tolerate a normal dose of a drug.

1.116   Which of the following statements about adverse drug reactions is correct?
A.   Long term adverse effects are easily recognised.
B.   Some drugs used for many years have subsequently been withdrawn.
C.   Clinical trials with patients are representative of the general population.
D.   All serious adverse effects are detected during clinical trials.

1.117 The intrinsic activity or efficacy of a drug is:
    A. a measure of its potency
    B. related to its maximal agonist effect
    C. related to its affinity for a receptor site
    D. restricted to describing antagonists
    E. the negative logarithm of the concentration producing half the maximum response.

1.118 Antagonists
    A. always bear an obvious structural relationship to agonists acting at the same receptor
    B. can only be discovered by random screening programmes
    C. are frequently active at more than one receptor site
    D. are invariably much larger molecules than agonists
    E. have a low affinity for the receptor and a high efficacy.

1.119 The pA_2 is:
    A. a measure of the potency of a competitive antagonist drug
    B. a measure of the potency of an agonist drug
    C. a measure of the intrinsic activity of an agonist drug
    D. a measure of the potency of a non-competitive antagonist drug.

1.120 Which of the following is not extractable from plants?
    A. atropine
    B. morphine
    C. digoxin
    D. cimetidine
    E. reserpine.

1.121 On the assumption that the passive transport of the non-ionised form of drugs determines the rate of their absorption, which of the following will be best absorbed in the small intestine?
    A. acetylsalicylic acid, pK_a 3.0
    B. phenytoin, pK_a 8.9
    C. phenobarbituric acid, pK_a 7.9
    D. salicylic acid, pK_a 3.0
    E. sulphadiazine, pK_a 6.5

1.122 Most quaternary nitrogen compounds do not penetrate the blood brain barrier because they:
    A. are very large molecules
    B. are negatively charged
    C. are poorly lipid soluble
    D. have hydrophilic groups
    E. do not have hydrophobic groups.

1.123 Chemicals may pass from maternal to foetal circulation if they have:
    A. molecular weight less than 300
    B. strong electropositive charge
    C. strong electronegative charge
    D. strong hydrophilic properties.

1.124   For optimal absorption after oral administration, a drug needs:
    A.   enteric coating
    B.   an ionised form
    C.   acid lability
    D.   lipid solubility.

1.125   Which of the following mechanisms is least likely to be involved in the biotransformation of drugs?
    A.   conjugation
    B.   oxidation
    C.   hydrolysis
    D.   esterification.

1.126   Biotransformation usually results in metabolites which, in comparison with the drug, have:
    A.   greater biological activity
    B.   greater water solubility
    C.   lower molecular weight
    D.   capacity for long storage in the body.

1.127   Which of the following enzymes is not important in drug biotransformation?
    A.   mixed function oxidase
    B.   cytochrome P450
    C.   monoamine oxidase
    D.   sulphonyl transferase
    E.   prostaglandin dehydrogenase.

1.128   Which of the following drugs does not induce hepatic drug metabolism?
    A.   phenytoin
    B.   carbamazepine
    C.   chloramphenicol
    D.   rifampicin
    E.   ethanol.

1.129   Which of the following drugs is not an enzyme inhibitor?
    A.   allopurinol
    B.   aspirin
    C.   atropine
    D.   α-methyldopa.

1.130   Which of the following is not a prodrug?
    A.   azathioprine
    B.   aspirin
    C.   cyclophosphamide
    D.   sulindac
    E.   cortisone.

1.131   Which of the following drugs does not have an active metabolite?
    A.   diazepam
    B.   phenacetin
    C.   aspirin
    D.   indomethacin
    E.   glutethimide.

1.132   Zero order kinetics apply when:
    A. the rate of drug elimination is constant, independent of the drug concentration in the body
    B. rapid enzyme induction increases drug clearance
    C. the rate of drug elimination decreases as the drug concentration in the body decreases
    D. none of the above.

1.133   Following a single oral dose of a drug, the point where the plasma concentration reaches a maximum is when:
    A. the rate of absorption is equal to the rate of elimination
    B. the rate of absorption is less than the rate of elimination
    C. the rate of absorption is greater than the rate of elimination
    D. elimination begins.

1.134   If a patient is receiving a drug by continuous intravenous infusion:
    A. 50% of the full clinical effect of the drug can be expected after a period equivalent to one half-life of the drug
    B. halving the concentration of the drug in the infused solution will reduce the half-life of elimination
    C. a steady state plasma level is achieved after a period equal to three to five half-lives of elimination
    D. none of the above.

1.135   The drug interaction of tetracycline and ferrous sulphate is most probably due to:
    A. displacement from plasma protein
    B. inhibition of metabolism
    C. induction of metabolism
    D. increased reabsorption from renal tubules
    E. decreased absorption from the gastrointestinal tract.

1.136   Metoclopramide can alter the plasma concentrations of other drugs because it:
    A. increases hepatic drug metabolism
    B. decreases gastric emptying
    C. decreases hepatic drug metabolism
    D. increases gastric emptying.

INCORRECT OPTION

1.137   Common binding forces in drug-receptor interactions are:
    A. electrostatic
    B. covalent
    C. hydrogen bonds
    D. van der Waals'.

1.138   Drug action may involve:
    A. alteration of normal physiological functions
    B. reversal of changes in body function resulting from disease.
    C. establishment of new functional properties of tissues
    D. exploitation of biochemical differences between host and parasite.

1.139   The advantages of administration by the intravenous route are:
     A.   higher initial blood levels
     B.   less risk of toxic effects
     C.   more accurate dosage possible
     D.   rapid onset of effects
     E.   large volumes can be administered.

1.140   Ferguson's thermodynamic activity of a drug:
     A.   is the same in all phases
     B.   is related to proportional saturation
     C.   can be measured in plasma
     D.   is equivalent to partial pressure for volatile drugs.

1.141   Serum protein binding of a drug:
     A.   is saturable
     B.   is greatest at high drug concentration
     C.   is reversible
     D.   may reduce the drug's metabolic rate.

1.142   Effective distribution of a drug in the body depends on:
     A.   degree of lipid solubility
     B.   degree of water solubility
     C.   degree of plasma protein binding
     D.   presence of an ionised from of drug.

1.143   In the body, drugs may be stored in:
     A.   liver
     B.   blood cells
     C.   bone
     D.   adipose tissue
     E.   saliva.

1.144   Serum protein binding of a drug may affect:
     A.   its rate of excretion
     B.   toxicity of another drug given concurrently
     C.   its route of administration
     D.   passage into the cerebrospinal fluid.

1.145   When a drug is given as a constant intravenous infusion:
     A.   steady state plasma concentration is achieved after a time period equivalent to between 3 and 5 plasma half-lives
     B.   the rate of infusion determines the steady state plasma concentration
     C.   plasma concentration achieves a value equivalent to half the final steady state concentration after a time period equivalent to one half-life
     D.   steady state plasma concentration is achieved only after liver enzyme induction has occurred.

1.146   Genetic factors account for variability in the metabolism of:
       A.   isoniazid
       B.   debrisoquine
       C.   metoprolol
       D.   procainamide
       E.   digoxin.

1.147   Glucuronide conjugation:
       A.   is influenced by the sex of the animals studied
       B.   may be altered by the presence of enzyme inducers or inhibitors
       C.   generates products which display equivalent physicochemical properties to the parent compound
       D.   is a synthetic reaction requiring energy and the transfer of a convenient moiety to the substrate.

MCQ

1.148   Herbal remedies may be effective because:
       i.   of the placebo effect
       ii.   they contain bacterial products which stimulate helper T-cells
       iii.   they contain pharmacologically active ingredients
       iv.   they pass along the bowel lumen without being absorbed.

1.149   Which of the following drugs is/are extracted from plants?
       i.   salbutamol
       ii.   atropine
       iii.   indomethacin
       iv.   morphine
       v.   propranolol.

1.150   Which of the following statements about drugs from plant sources is/are true?
       i.   Cocaine is a central nervous system stimulant.
       ii.   Extract of belladonna is used in gastrointestinal medicines.
       iii.   Bark from the cinchona tree contains quinine.
       iv.   Heroin is found in the opium poppy.
       v.   Stramonium contains cardiac stimulants.

1.151   Which of the following statements about adverse drug reactions is/are correct?
       i.   Notification to the Department of adverse drug reactions is compulsory.
       ii.   The Australian Drug Evaluation Committee assesses a new drug's safety and efficacy.
       iii.   Adverse drug reaction monitoring is a function of the State Department of Health.
       iv.   Most drugs marketed in Australia prior to 1969 have not been evaluated retrospectively.
       v.   Medications purchased 'over the counter' at pharmacies are devoid of adverse effects.

1.152   The therapeutic index of a drug is:
     i.   constant over all doses for all adverse effects
     ii.   an index of safety for the specified drug
     iii. the same, regardless of the route of administration
     iv. the separation between the therapeutic and unwanted effects
     v.   the profitability prediction of that drug.

1.153   An idiosyncratic drug reaction is:
     i.   not dose-related
     ii.   a rare event
     iii. due to factors which increase host susceptibility
     iv. seldom of clinical significance
     v.   more frequently found in feeble minded patients.

1.154   Tolerance:
     i.   is a condition of decreased responsiveness acquired on repeated exposure to a drug
     ii.   developed to rapid, repeated exposure to a drug is known as anaphylaxis
     iii. may have a pharmacokinetic and/or a pharmacodynamic basis
     iv. causes the patient to respond to smaller and smaller doses of the drug
     v.   is transmitted by T4 and T8 subsets of lymphocytes.

1.155   Competitive antagonism exists when:
     i.   the agonist and the antagonist have affinity for the same receptor
     ii.   the antagonism may be overcome by increasing the dose of agonist
     iii. only the agonist has appreciable efficacy
     iv. the antagonist acts through different but not independent receptors
     v.   the antagonist is more potent than the agonist.

1.156   The drugs most suitable for transcutaneous administration:
     i.   are effective in daily dose of 100-500 mg
     ii.   have molecular weight of up to 2000
     iii. are prodrugs
     iv. are subject to variable first-pass metabolism.

1.157   When reliable absorption of a drug is desired over a prolonged period of time, the best administration procedure/s is/are:
     i.   oral ingestion
     ii.   intramuscular injection of the drug in suspension
     iii. intravenous injection of an insoluble form of the drug
     iv. subcutaneous implantation of a solid drug pellet.

1.158   Which of the following are potential sites for drug biotransformation?
     i.   plasma
     ii.   liver
     iii. intestine
     iv. lung.

1.159   The half-life of elimination of a drug
      i.   is inversely related to the clearance of the drug
      ii.   is a determinant of the loading dose of the drug
      iii. may be calculated from the rate constant for the process of elimination
      iv. is equivalent to the time taken to achieve steady state plasma concentration.

1.160   Microsomal mixed function oxidases may be inhibited by:
      i.   allopurinol
      ii.   chloramphenicol
      iii. cimetidine
      iv. phenytoin
      v.   rifampicin.

1.161   The clearance of a drug is related to:
      i.   bioavailability
      ii.   half-life
      iii. rate of absorption
      iv. volume of distribution
      v.   partition coefficient.

1.162   For a drug infused rapidly i.v., if the plot of log plasma concentration against time has two linear components:
      i.   the initial phase is the absorption phase
      ii.   the existence of a two-compartment model is suggested
      iii. the second phase represents a zero-order elimination
      iv. the model is behaving as a single compartment during the final phase of elimination
      v.   the distribution phase has second order kinetics.

ASSERTION/REASON

1.163   Pharmacologically active alternative therapies may be useful therapeutic agents **BECAUSE** pharmacologically active alternative therapies are non-toxic.

1.164   Ionised drug molecules do not diffuse through cell membranes **BECAUSE** ionised drug molecules are larger than non-ionised drug molecules.

1.165   Intravenous injection of drugs will produce higher plasma concentrations than oral administration **BECAUSE** the dose used for intravenous injection is always larger than that administered orally.

1.166   The degree of protein binding may alter the duration of action of a drug **BECAUSE** protein binding retards renal excretion.

1.167   Biotransformation of a drug always gives rise to a less toxic substance **BECAUSE** biotransformation always reduces the size of the molecule.

1.168 Sulindac is a prodrug **BECAUSE** sulindac has greater biological activity than its metabolites.

1.169 Drugs can be protected from first pass hepatic metabolism by sublingual administration **BECAUSE** sublingual administration spares drugs from acid digestion.

1.170 Concomitant administration of diazepam and cimetidine results in elevated plasma diazepam concentrations **BECAUSE** diazepam and cimetidine compete for the same metabolic pathway.

ANSWERS

1.1	T	1.35	F	1.69	T	1.103	T	1.137	B
1.2	T	1.36	T	1.70	T	1.104	F	1.138	C
1.3	T	1.37	F	1.71	F	1.105	F	1.139	B
1.4	T	1.38	T	1.72	T	1.106	T	1.140	D
1.5	F	1.39	T	1.73	T	1.107	T	1.141	B
1.6	T	1.40	F	1.74	F	1.108	F	1.142	D
1.7	T	1.41	T	1.75	T	1.109	T	1.143	E
1.8	T	1.42	F	1.76	T	1.110	F	1.144	C
1.9	T	1.43	T	1.77	F	1.111	F	1.145	D
1.10	F	1.44	F	1.78	F	1.112	F	1.146	E
1.11	T	1.45	T	1.79	T	1.113	F	1.147	C
1.12	F	1.46	F	1.80	F	1.114	F	1.148	B
1.13	F	1.47	F	1.81	F	1.115	A	1.149	C
1.14	F	1.48	T	1.82	T	1.116	B	1.150	A
1.15	T	1.49	F	1.83	T	1.117	B	1.151	C
1.16	F	1.50	F	1.84	T	1.118	C	1.152	C
1.17	T	1.51	T	1.85	T	1.119	A	1.153	A
1.18	T	1.52	T	1.86	F	1.120	D	1.154	B
1.19	T	1.53	T	1.87	F	1.121	B	1.155	A
1.20	T	1.54	F	1.88	F	1.122	C	1.156	D
1.21	T	1.55	F	1.89	F	1.123	A	1.157	C
1.22	F	1.56	F	1.90	T	1.124	D	1.158	E
1.23	T	1.57	T	1.91	F	1.125	D	1.159	B
1.24	T	1.58	F	1.92	F	1.126	B	1.160	A
1.25	F	1.59	F	1.93	F	1.127	E	1.161	C
1.26	F	1.60	F	1.94	T	1.128	C	1.162	C
1.27	T	1.61	T	1.95	F	1.129	C	1.163	C
1.28	F	1.62	F	1.96	F	1.130	B	1.164	C
1.29	T	1.63	T	1.97	T	1.131	D	1.165	C
1.30	T	1.64	F	1.98	F	1.132	A	1.166	A
1.31	F	1.65	T	1.99	F	1.133	A	1.167	E
1.32	T	1.66	T	1.100	F	1.134	C	1.168	C
1.33	T	1.67	F	1.101	F	1.135	E	1.169	B
1.34	F	1.68	T	1.102	T	1.136	D	1.170	A

2 Molecular Pharmacology

TRUE / FALSE

2.1   The activity of the majority of drug molecules can be predicted with certainty by examining conformational structure.

2.2   Positional isomers are molecules that differ in a position of a substituent, but still have the same chemical formulae.

2.3   Optical isomers differ only in their colour.

2.4   In drugs which contain a symmmetric carbon atom, one optical isomer is always more biologically active than the other.

2.5   Bioisosteres are functional groups which can be used in a molecularly modified drug to replace a certain functional group in the original drug, so that the modified drug acquires antagonist properties at the receptor site.

2.6   Bioisosteric replacement of a functional group in a drug molecule can lead to a more selective agent.

2.7   An important consideration for isosteric replacement in drug molecules is that the new drug molecule should posses the same total charge in order to interact with the same receptor site.

2.8   The lowest energy conformation of a flexible drug molecule is the most active conformation at the target receptor.

2.9   Structural similarities between a series of agonists and antagonists do not necessarily mean that both classes of substances are likely to act at the same receptor.

2.10   An acetyl substituent is necessary for a drug to have similar pharmacological properties to acetylcholine.

2.11   Pharmacological activity in the homologous series of alkyl alcohols increases with the size of the alkyl group until a critical cut-off point is reached.

2.12   A drug which is ionised will not readily cross the blood brain barrier.

2.13   Steroids contain trans-fused cyclohexane rings held in the chair conformation.

2.14   Rotation about carbon-carbon double bonds is sufficiently rapid at body temperature so that cis and trans isomers have similar pharmacological activity.

2.15   Drugs with cis-substituted double bonds are usually rapidly isomerised in the body.

2.16   Hydrophobic substituents can increase the affinity of a drug for the receptor.

2.17   "Antimetabolite" drugs are designed to resemble a normal substrate or metabolite of a key enzymic pathway.

2.18   In drug molecules, a compound with an alcohol substituent is always more active than the corresponding ester.

2.19   Similar odours may be evoked by substances of vastly different composition, and totally different odours may be produced by related chemicals.

2.20   Simple chemicals with a tertiary carbon atom often have a camphoraceous odour.

2.21   The formula below represents 4 separate enantiomers.

CORRECT OPTION:

2.22

I   II

The formulae I and II represent:
   A.   the same optical isomer of one compound
   B.   different optical isomers of one compound
   C.   the same compound which is optically active
   D.   two quite different chemical substances.

INCORRECT OPTION

2.23 In designing new drugs, the conformation of a flexible agonist may be restricted by:
    A. introducing unsaturation
    B. incorporating an alicyclic ring
    C. incorporating a heterocyclic ring
    D. isosteric replacement
    E. adding bulky substituents.

2.24 A drug may be designed to inhibit a specific enzyme by acting as a:
    A. transition state analogue
    B. substrate analogue
    C. cofactor analogue
    D. suicide substrate
    E. false transmitter.

2.25 With regard to taste:
    A. Aspartame is sweeter than sucrose.
    B. Bitter tastes are most easily sensed at the sides of the tongue.
    C. Highly ionised inorganic salts of low molecular weight usually evoke a salty taste.
    D. Lipid solubility can contribute to the sour taste of organic acids.
    E. Some substances can evoke different tastes according to their concentrations.

2.26 With regard to taste:
    A. The ability of a compound to participate in hydrogen bonding is an important prerequisite for it to taste sweet.
    B. Aqueous sulphuric acid has a sour taste.
    C. Many alkaloids are bitter-tasting.
    D. Pure water is always tasteless.
    E. Some substances taste both bitter and sweet.

ANSWERS

2.1	F	2.7	T	2.13	T	2.19	T	2.25	B
2.2	T	2.8	F	2.14	F	2.20	T	2.26	D
2.3	F	2.9	T	2.15	F	2.21	T		
2.4	F	2.10	F	2.16	T	2.22	B		
2.5	F	2.11	T	2.17	T	2.23	D		
2.6	T	2.12	T	2.18	F	2.24	E		

3 Central Nervous System

TRUE / FALSE

3.1 The ratio of ATP to neurotransmitter is the same in all synaptic vesicles so far studied.

3.2 Most neurones in the central nervous system release peptides as transmitters.

3.3 When different peptides co-exist in a neurone, they always derive from a common precursor.

3.4 Drugs that inhibit transmitter inactivation will usually produce convulsions in experimental animals.

3.5 Convulsant drugs stimulate glial cells.

3.6 Transmitters mediate synaptic transmission between neurones and glial cells.

3.7 Blocking the postsynaptic action of a transmitter will have a similiar effect to blocking its synthesis.

3.8 The potency of central nervous system depressant drugs in a homologous series varies directly with the molecular weight.

3.9 Many hallucinogens have structures resembling natural neurotransmitters.

3.10 Ascending paralysis following administration of a neurotoxin is unequivocal evidence for a central site of action.

3.11 Neuroleptanalgesia is induced by the combination of a potent narcotic analgesic and a butyrophenone antipsychotic drug.

3.12 General anaesthetics are thought to reduce the fluidity of mammalian cell membranes.

3.13 Induction of anaesthesia using inhalational anaesthetic agents is rapid if the blood/gas partition coefficient of the agent is high.

3.14 Hypercarbia lowers the threshold for the occurrence of cardiac arrhythmias during general anaesthesia.

3.15 V The second gas effect allows a lower than normal concentration of oxygen to be inspired during a mask induction without hypoxaemia occurring.

19

3.16   The potency of a general anaesthetic gas varies directly with the ratio of its saturated vapour pressure to the partial pressure at which it is used.

3.17   The residual effects of general anaesthetics on psychomotor performance may persist for 48 hours.

3.18   Chronic exposure to trace concentrations of anaesthetic agents is reported to increase the risk of spontaneous abortion among exposed females.

3.19   Alphaxalone is a steroidal intravenous anaesthetic.

3.20   Halothane produces a dose-dependent bradycardia.

3.21 V Induction of anaesthesia with halothane will be prolonged in the hypovolaemic patient.

3.22   The hypotensive effect of halothane is associated with a reduction of cardiac output.

3.23   Nitrous oxide is narcotic when its partial pressure equals its saturated vapour pressure.

3.24   The addition of nitrous oxide lowers the minimum alveolar concentration of the volatile anaesthetic agents.

3.25   Nitrous oxide can safely be administered to a patient with pneumothorax.

3.26   Addition of nitrous oxide to a halothane anaesthetic will cause an increase in blood pressure.

3.27 V Adrenaline tartrate can safely be administered to a dog anaesthetised with enflurane.

3.28   Patients must usually take benzodiazepines for at least one week before clinically useful anti-anxiety effects are observed.

3.29   The absorption of diazepam is enhanced if ethanol is consumed concomitantly.

3.30   Benzodiazepines may, in some patients, induce violent behaviour.

3.31   Benzodiazepines increase the affinity of GABA for GABA binding sites in rat brain membranes.

3.32   Benzodiazepines increase the frequency of opening of chloride channels activated by GABA.

3.33   Benzodiazepines block GABA release.

3.34   Barbiturates and benzodiazepines potentiate the actions of glycine as an inhibitory neurotransmitter.

3.35   Barbiturates potentiate GABA action.

3.36   Barbiturates inhibit glutamate release.

3.37   Barbiturates increase the number of GABA binding sites.

3.38   Barbiturates taken regularly over a period of weeks will induce hepatic microsomal enzymes.

3.39   Parkinson's disease is characterised by an increase in brain monoamine oxidase levels.

3.40   In Parkinson's disease, levodopa therapy is more effective for hypokinesia than for tremor.

3.41   There is no decline in the efficacy of levodopa in Parkinson's disease, even after several years of use.

4.42   Patients who take bromocriptine may develop galactorrhoea.

3.43   Tyrosine is an effective treatment for Parkinson's disease.

3.44   All drugs effective in the control of epilepsy produce sedation.

3.45   Anticonvulsants may act by inhibiting the inactivation of an inhibitory neurotransmitter.

3.46   Anticonvulsants, such as barbiturates and benzodiazepines, act by enhancing inhibitory synaptic transmission.

3.47   Phenytoin plasma concentrations correlate well with therapeutic effects and toxicity.

3.48   Phenytoin is extensively metabolised by hepatic microsomal enzymes.

3.49   Tetrahydrocannabinol may precipitate fitting in an epileptic patient.

3.50   Neuroleptics are the drugs of choice for the treatment of psychoneuroses.

3.51   All clinically useful neuroleptics are potent antagonists at dopamine D_2 receptors.

3.52   Butyrophenones act as muscle relaxants.

3.53   Tolerance develops to the antipsychotic effects of the butyrophenones.

3.54   Antimuscarinic agents exacerbate neuroleptic-induced acute dystonia.

3.55   Benztropine exacerbates neuroleptic induced Parkinsonian-like side effects.

3.56   The symptoms of haloperidol-induced tardive dyskinesia can be ameliorated by increasing the dose of haloperidol.

3.57   Chlorpromazine increases the concentration of prolactin in the blood of normal subjects.

3.58   Hypersensitivity to chlorpromazine may be aggravated by ultraviolet light.

3.59   A hypertensive crisis, due to increased levels of circulating catecholamines, is a major side effect of tricyclic antidepressants.

3.60   The release of enkephalins is not dependent upon calcium ions.

3.61   Opiate receptors are found only in the central nervous system.

3.62V   The subcutaneous administration of a small dose of morphine to the cat lowers its body temperature.

3.63   Etorphine is a powerful opiate antagonist.

3.64   Pentazocine is a useful analgesic with mixed agonist-antagonist activity.

3.65   Morphine binds to a single population of opiate binding sites in the brain.

3.66   Radioligand binding studies with opiates cannot differentiate between agonists and antagonists.

3.67   Opiate receptor agonists stimulate adenyl cyclase activity.

3.68   Enkephalins are non-addictive analgesics.

3.69   β-Endorphin is the major precursor of leu-enkephalin.

3.70   After release, peptides are inactivated by a specific uptake process.

3.71   Leu-enkephalin appears to act as an inhibitory transmitter in the central nervous system.

3.72   The precursor molecule for leu-enkephalin is pro-opiocortin.

3.73   Substance P is an opiate receptor agonist.

3.74   Capsaicin antagonises the post synaptic actions of substance P on spinal neurones.

3.75   Specific peptides produce REM and slow wave sleep.

3.76   The endorphins are non-addictive analgesics.

3.77   Enkephalins and substance P are involved in the perception of pain.

3.78   Acupuncture analgesia may involve activation of endogenous opiate systems.

3.79   Glycine is produced by decarboxylation of glutamate.

3.80   Glycine and GABA are excitatory transmitters in the spinal cord.

3.81   Glycine and aspartate are important transmitters in the spinal cord.

3.82   Strychnine produces convulsions by antagonising the action of glycine in the spinal cord.

3.83   Tetanus toxin prevents the release of glycine.

3.84   Control of motor function involves synaptic inhibition that can be blocked by tetanus toxin.

3.85   Taurine is the most abundant amino acid in infant brain.

3.86 Taurine may be an important excitatory transmitter in the cerebellum.

3.87 Taurine-induced inhibition can be antagonised by strychnine.

3.88 GABA is synthesised in the nervous system by enzymatic decarboxylation of glutamic acid.

3.89 GABA receptors in the forebrain influence sympathetic cardiovascular activity.

3.90 Endogenous inhibitors influence the activity of GABA receptors and ionophores

3.91 Anxiety may be associated with an increased activity of GABA receptors.

3.92 A drug which blocks the uptake of GABA would be expected to have anticonvulsant properties.

3.93 Agents which block GABA synthesis are tranquillisers.

3.94 Regional brain levels of GABA are of the same order of magnitude as those of dopamine.

3.95 The loss of GABA neurones in Huntington's disease is accompanied by a net loss in the number of GABA receptors.

3.96 Glutamate receptors may be classified on the basis of the actions of the selective agonists kainate, quisqualate and NMDA.

3.97 Glutamate is inactivated by uptake processes in neurones and glia.

3.98 Glutamate and kainate can kill glial cells.

3.99 Glutamate release can be potentiated by baclofen, a drug used to treat spasticity.

3.100 Noradrenaline and dopamine are the major inhibitory transmitters in the central nervous system.

3.101 Dopamine turnover may be assessed indirectly by measuring the metabolites DOPAC and HVA in the urine.

3.102 The activity of dopamine terminals in the corpus striatum is modulated by an excitatory cholinergic influence.

3.103V Apomorphine is an effective analgesic in the dog.

3.104 Dopamine antagonists act on the tuberoinfundibular system to cause a marked rise in prolactin levels.

3.105 6-Hydroxydopamine exerts its action by the generation of a false transmitter after enzymatic decarboxylation.

3.106 6-Hydroxydopamine is a selective neurotoxin for dopamine and noradrenaline neuronal systems.

3.107 Huntington's disease can be treated using dopamine precursors.

3.108   (+)-Amphetamine releases "newly-synthesised" stores of dopamine.

3.109   Picrotoxin causes CNS excitation by inhibiting dopamine systems.

3.110   Caffeine potentiates the inhibitory action of noradrenaline in the central nervous system.

3.111   p-Chlorophenylalanine can block the synthesis of 5-hydroxytryptamine in CNS neurones.

3.112   Many hallucinogenic drugs are structurally related to 5-hydroxytryptamine .

3.113   The inhibition by 5-hydroxytryptamine of lateral geniculate nucleus neuronal firing is due to an action at presynaptic inhibitory receptors.

3.114   Acetylcholine is the transmitter at most synapses in the brain.

3.115   Acetylcholine neurones are intrinsic to the cerebral cortex.

3.116   Presynaptic muscarinic receptors have been shown to exist on cholinergic nerves.

3.117   Vasoactive intestinal peptide greatly increases the affinity of some cholinergic receptors for acetylcholine.

3.118   Acetylcholine can activate nicotinic receptors in the spinal cord, thalamus and cerebral cortex.

3.119   In the central nervous system, both nicotinic and muscarinic receptors for acetylcholine have been found.

3.120   Hemicholinium blocks acetylcholine synthesis by inhibiting choline acetyltransferase.

3.121   Kainic acid lesions in the central nervous system cause an almost total disappearance of histamine-sensitive adenyl cyclase.

3.122   Kainate lesions are similar to those found in certain neurodegenerative diseases.

3.123   Central nervous system synaptosomal histamine is synthesised by histamine-N-methyltransferase.

3.124   Histamine-sensitive adenyl cyclase in the central nervous system is probably linked to histamine H_2 receptors.

3.125   All histamine in the central nervous system is contained within mast cells.

3.126   Carnosine is the main neurotransmitter involved in processing taste information in the nucleus of the tractus solitarius.

3.127   Inhibition of cyclic AMP phosphodiesterase is no longer considered the sole mechanism of action giving rise to the central effects of theophylline.

CORRECT OPTION

3.128 The specialised structure of brain capillaries is induced by:
    A.   astrocyte influence
    B.   blood-borne factors
    C.   ionic changes in extracellular fluid
    D.   neuronal activity.

3.129 The blood brain barrier is primarily:
    A.   a passive restriction on the entry of pharmacologically active substances from blood to brain
    B.   a vascular barrier that is selectively permeable and involved with the active transport and secretion of compounds between brain and blood
    C.   a barrier protecting the immature brain *in utero*
    D.   a feature of the brain capillaries of the primitive vertebrate nervous system, subsequently lost during evolution.

3.130 Polar drug metabolites formed in the central nervous system and lacking specific carriers across the blood brain barrier:
    A.   accumulate in the extracellular space until absorbed by neurones
    B.   diffuse into the cerebrospinal fluid and are cleared from the brain
    C.   poison the brain
    D.   are taken up by macrophages.

3.131 Which of the following properties would you expect a centrally active drug to possess?
    A.   strong binding to plasma proteins
    B.   an ionised form
    C.   a high hexane/water partition coefficient
    D.   a high chemical reactivity
    E.   molecular weight greater than 1500.

3.132 In general, the most important factor influencing drug entry into the brain is:
    A.   lipid solubility
    B.   water solubility
    C.   molecular weight
    D.   molecular shape.

3.133 Tetrodotoxin can be used to count voltage-gated sodium channels because:
    A.   it binds irreversibly to voltage-gated sodium channels
    B.   its interaction with voltage-gated sodium channels can be described by first order kinetics
    C.   it is water soluble
    D.   its binding is voltage dependent
    E.   it is a non-protein molecule.

3.134   The major inhibitory transmitter in the brain is:
      A.   glycine
      B.   noradrenaline
      C.   GABA
      D.   glutamic acid.

3.135   For compounds acting as inhalation anaesthetics:
      A.   within a homologous series, potency generally decreases gradually as the length of the carbon chain increases
      B.   olefins are less potent then the corresponding paraffins
      C.   halogen substitution of parrafins generally increases potency
      D.   alcohols are much more potent than the corresponding ethers.

3.136   Induction of anaesthesia with inhalational anaesthetic agents is:
      A.   hastened if ventilation is decreased
      B.   hastened if cardiac output is increased
      C.   hastened if high concentrations of nitrous oxide are inspired with the potent anaesthetic agent
      D.   rapid if the anaesthetic agent has a high blood/gas partition coefficient
      E.   rapid if the anaesthetic agents as a high oil/gas partition coefficient.

3.137   Which of the following volatile anaesthetic agents has been most commonly associated with hepatotoxicity?
      A.   halothane
      B.   isoflurane
      C.   methoxyflurane
      D.   enflurane
      E.   trichloroethylene.

3.138   Nephrotoxicity is dose-dependent with:
      A.   halothane
      B.   isoflurane
      C.   methoxyflurane
      D.   enflurane
      E.   trichloroethylene.

3.139V Saffan:
      A.   is a barbiturate induction agent
      B.   can be safely administered to the dog
      C.   produces anaesthesia when administered subcutaneously
      D.   causes dose-dependent hypertension
      E.   has a higher incidence of anaphylactoid reactions than thiopentone sodium.

3.140   A.   GABA-transaminase catalyses the synthesis of GABA.
      B.   Neuroleptic agents are the treatment of choice for neuroses.
      C.   Benzodiazepines are effective in the treatment of epilepsy.
      D.   Tyrosine hydroxylase inhibitors are effective adjuncts to levodopa therapy.
      E.   Tranylcypromine is a tricyclic antidepressant.

3.141   Diazepam is most likely to cause:
    A.   urinary retention
    B.   severe diarrhoea
    C.   physical dependence
    D.   acute dystonia.

3.142   Symptoms of withdrawal following sudden cessation of benzodiazepines usually last for:
    A.   6 to 8 hours
    B.   24 to 48 hours
    C.   3 to 5 days
    D.   7 to 10 days
    E.   3 to 4 weeks.

3.143V Which of the following is not used as a sedative-hypnotic drug?
    A.   chloral hydrate
    B.   sodium bromide
    C.   pentobarbitone
    D.   xylazine
    E.   phenytoin.

3.144   MPTP is thought to cause Parkinsonism by:
    A.   destroying fibres of the rubrospinal tract
    B.   destroying cells in the substantia nigra pars compacta
    C.   depleting catecholamine stores in nerve terminals
    D.   blocking the synthesis of dopamine
    E.   increasing cholinergic drive to the substantia nigra.

3.145   Sodium valproate is:
    A.   a general anaesthetic
    B.   an anticonvulsant
    C.   a local anaesthetic
    D.   a sedative-hypnotic
    E.   an antidepressant.

3.146   The increased abnormal involuntary movements induced by levodopa in some patients with Parkinson's disease are called:
    A.   akinesias
    B.   ramifications
    C.   dyskinesias
    D.   hypertonicities
    E.   tardive dyskinesias.

3.147   Side effects of phenytoin include :
    A.   drowsiness, headache, ataxia
    B.   ataxia, skin eruptions, nystagmus, paraesthesia
    C.   gum hyperplasia, mild polyneuritis, hirsutism
    D.   photophobia, skin eruptions, bone marrow depression
    E.   hair loss, abdominal cramps, diarrhoea.

3.148   Neuroleptic drugs may produce extrapyramidal neurological signs because they:
    A.   deplete stores of noradrenaline in the substantia nigra
    B.   antagonise the central effects of acetylcholine
    C.   suppress inhibitory reflex pathways in the spinal cord
    D.   are dopamine receptor antagonists
    E.   none of the above.

3.149   The most appropriate drug for the long-term treatment of schizophrenia is:
    A.   diazepam
    B.   aspirin
    C.   amitriptyline
    D.   chlorpromazine
    E.   bromocriptine.

3.150   Which of the following most accurately describes the action of haloperidol?
    A.   blockade of dopamine receptors in the central nervous system
    B.   blockade of dopamine and noradrenaline receptors in the central nervous system
    C.   blockade of noradrenaline receptors in the central nervous system.

3.151   Neuroleptanalgesia is a therapeutic procedure utilising the administration of which of the following combinations?
    A.   heroin and diazepam
    B.   chlorpromazine and aspirin
    C.   droperidol and fentanyl
    D.   haloperidol and naloxone
    E.   droperidol and diazepam.

3.152   Which of the following is the most appropriate treatment for endogenous depression?
    A.   chloral hydrate
    B.   chlorpromazine
    C.   amitriptyline
    D.   vitamin C
    E.   diazepam.

3.153   Which of the following antidepressants is a monoamine oxidase inhibitor at normal clinical doses?
    A.   tranylcypromine
    B.   mianserin
    C.   imipramine
    D.   (+)-amphetamine
    E.   amitriptyline.

3.154   Which of the following antidepressants is the most sedative?
    A.   tranylcypromine
    B.   amitriptyline
    C.   desipramine
    D.   doxepin
    E.   protriptyline.

3.155   A patient on medication presents with the following drug-induced side effects: manic excitement, dry mouth, constipation, tachycardia, excessive sweating and urinary retention. Which of the following drugs is most likely to be responsible?
    A.   chlorpromazine
    B.   amitriptyline
    C.   homatropine
    D.   diazepam
    E.   apomorphine.

3.156   Which of the following foodstuffs is not contraindicated in patients taking tranylcypromine?
    A.   beer
    B.   red wine
    C.   red meat
    D.   chicken liver
    E.   pickled herring.

3.157   The major active constituent of *Papaver somniferum* is:
    A.   heroin
    B.   Δ-9-tetrahydrocannabinol
    C.   morphine
    D.   dihydromorphinone.

3.158   Which of the following peptides is not contained in the amino acid sequence of pro-opiocortin?
    A.   α-melanocyte stimulating hormone
    B.   adrenocorticotrophic hormone
    C.   leu-enkephalin
    D.   met-enkephalin
    E.   β-endorphin.

3.159   Which of the following enzymes does not perform post-translational processing of one or more neuropeptides?
    A.   trypsin-like enzymes
    B.   carboxypeptidase-B-like enzymes
    C.   angiotensin converting enzyme
    D.   enkephalinase.

3.160   Which of the following has the lowest analgesic potency after i.v. administration?
    A.   β-endorphin
    B.   morphine
    C.   met-enkephalin
    D.   ala-2-met-enkephalin
    E.   levorphanol.

3.161   Which of the following statements about dopamine pathways in the brain is correct?
    A.   The nucleus accumbens in the limbic system is innervated from cell bodies in the substantia nigra.
    B.   The nigrostriatal pathway consists of cell bodies in the caudate nucleus projecting axons to the substantia nigra.
    C.   The nigrostriatal pathway consists of cell bodies in the substantia nigra, projecting axons to various nuclei including the caudate nucleus.
    D.   Dopamine neurones project from the cerebellar cortex to the deep cerebellar nuclei.

3.162   Which of the following enzymes is rate limiting in the synthesis of dopamine?
    A.   DOPA decarboxylase
    B.   phenylethanolamine-N-methyl transferase
    C.   tyrosine hydroxylase
    D.   monoamine oxidase
    E.   dopamine-β-hydroxylase.

3.163   Dopamine neurones can be destroyed by:
        A.   6-hydroxydopamine
        B.   L-DOPA
        C.   noradrenaline
        D.   GABA
        E.   apomorphine.

3.164   The treatment of choice for the movement problems associated with Huntington's disease is:
        A.   levodopa
        B.   bromocriptine
        C.   apomorphine
        D.   haloperidol.

3.165   Bromocriptine:
        A.   is predominantly an antimuscarinic
        B.   can cause severe cardiovascular side effects
        C.   is a precursor for dopamine
        D.   can cause tardive dyskinesia
        E.   is a directly acting D_2 dopamine receptor agonist.

3.166   Which of the following drugs is most likely to be used to treat hyperprolactinaemia?
        A.   metoclopramide
        B.   bromocriptine
        C.   chlorpromazine
        D.   baclofen
        E.   carbamazepine.

3.167   Amino acids are:
        A.   transported across the blood brain barrier by one single carrier and are maintained at equal concentration in extracellular fluid.
        B.   all neurotransmitters and hence blood-borne amino acids are excluded form the extracellular space
        C.   transported across the blood brain barrier by several carriers and are subsequently subject to various uptake processes by neurones and glia
        D.   subject to passive diffusion into the extracellular space and then are actively taken up by neurones and glia.

3.168   The major postsynaptic effect of GABA in the central nervous system is:
        A.   hyperpolarisation by an increased chloride conductance
        B.   hypopolarisation by an increased chloride conductance
        C.   hyperpolarisation by altering sodium and potassium conductance
        D.   hypopolarisation by altering sodium and potassium conductance
        E.   a selective block of any increase in sodium conductance with little change in membrane potential.

3.169   GABA or GABA-mimetics administered intracerebroventricularly will:
        A.   enhance growth hormone release
        B.   inhibit growth hormone release
        C.   have no effect on growth hormone release.

3.170   The transmitter at "purinergic nerves" is proposed to be:
      A.   inosine
      B.   cytosine
      C.   adenosine triphosphate
      D.   caffeine
      E.   adenine.

3.171   Purines can produce muscle relaxation by:
      A.   blocking the synthesis of acetylcholine in cholinergic nerves
      B.   blocking acetylcholine receptors at the neuromuscular junction
      C.   depressing transmission at central synapses
      D.   reducing blood flow to skeletal muscle
      E.   blocking action potentials in motor nerves.

3.172   Which of the following is a 5-hydroxytryptamine receptor agonist in brain tissue?
      A.   LSD
      B.   reserpine
      C.   p-chlorophenylalanine
      D.   allylglycine.

3.173-3.175

3.173   amitriptyline

3.174   reserpine

3.175   diazepam

For each of the drugs listed above, indicate whether it is most likely to cause:

      A.   dry mouth
      B.   suicidal depression
      C.   physical dependence
      D.   tardive dyskinesia.

3.176-3.179

3.176   diazepam

3.177   trimethadione

3.178   phenytoin

3.179   carbamazepine

For each of the drugs listed above, indicate whether it:

      A.   causes gastrointestinal irritation
      B.   is structurally related to the tricyclic antidepressants
      C.   is of value for the treatment of absence seizures
      D.   is effective for the immediate suppression of a series of grand mal convulsions, but only when given intravenously.

3.180-3.181

3.180   grand mal seizures are likely during withdrawal after chronic administration

3.181   is liable to produce a paranoid psychosis

For each of the statements above, indicate whether it applies to:

A.   dextropropoxyphene
B.   (+)-amphetamine
C.   Δ-9-tetrahydrocannabinol
D.   quinalbarbitone.

3.182-3.183

3.182   produces tardive dyskinesia

3.183   is liable to produce physical dependency

For each of the statements above, indicate whether it applies to:

A.   amylobarbitone
B.   pilocarpine
C.   imipramine
D.   aspirin
E.   haloperidol.

3.184-3.187

3.184   methoxyflurane

3.185   cyclopropane

3.186   trichloroethylene

3.187   halothane

For each of the drugs listed above, indicate whether it is:

A.   an ether
B.   a halogenated hydrocarbon
C.   an inorganic oxide
D.   an alicyclic hydrocarbon.

3.188 - 3.192

3.188   deprenyl

3.189   carbidopa

3.190   benztropine

3.191   bromocriptine

3.192   levodopa

All of the drugs listed above are used in the treatment of Parkinson's disease. For each of these, indicate the most appropriate description of its mode of action:

A.   directly acting dopamine D_2 receptor agonist
B.   antimuscarinic
C.   peripheral decarboxylase inhibitor
D.   precursor of dopamine
E.   monoamine oxidase inhibitor.

3.193 - 3.196

3.193   psychomotor epilepsy

3.194   "absences"

3.195   status epilepticus

3.196   grand mal epilepsy

For each of the types of epilepsy listed above, indicate the most appropriate treatment:

A. phenobarbitone
B. diazepam (i.v.)
C. ethosuxamide
D. carbamazepine.

3.197 - 3.198

3.197   desipramine

3.198   mianserin

For each of the drugs listed above, indicate whether it:

A.   predominantly inhibits noradrenaline uptake
B.   predominantly inhibits dopamine uptake
C.   predominantly inhibits 5-hydroxytryptamine uptake
D.   none of the above.

3.199 - 3.201

3.199   most potent agonist

3.200   agonist and antagonist

3.201   pure antagonist

For each of the descriptions of opiate analgesic activity above, indicate whether it most appropriately applies to:

A.   the N-allyl derivative of pethidine
B.   etorphine
C.   levorphanol
D.   naloxone
E.   pentazocine.

INCORRECT OPTION

3.202   Central nervous system raphe nuclei:
A.   axons project to brain stem regions
B.   axons contain aromatic L-amino acid decarboxylase
C.   axons are tryptaminergic
D.   cell bodies possess receptors for 5-hydroxytryptamine
E.   stimulation results in excitation of lateral geniculate nucleus neurones.

3.203V Minimum alveolar concentration (MAC):
A.   of a particular anaesthetic agent is decreased in the presence of narcotic analgesics
B.   falls with increasing age
C.   is decreased by shock
D.   is less for methoxyflurane than for halothane
E.   is the same as the value needed to produce surgical anaesthesia.

3.204V Isoflurane:
A.   produces a faster induction and recovery than halothane
B.   is a structural isomer of enflurane
C.   does not depress respiration
D.   potentiates the effects of non-depolarising muscle relaxants
E.   can be safely administered to an animal undergoing electrocautery.

3.205   Chloral hydrate:
A.   is rapidly reduced in the body to trichlorethanol
B.   has a foul, bitter taste
C.   is useful for patients with gastric ulcers
D.   potentiates the action of ethanol
E.   can produce dependency.

3.206   A.   Benzodiazepines have a wider safety margin than most other hypnotics.

            B.   Cases of barbiturate poisoning should be treated with a central nervous system stimulant to counteract central depression.

            C.   Ethanol potentiates the action of chloral hydrate.

            D.   Cessation of barbiturate treatment disturbs the ratio of REM to non-REM sleep.

            E.   Hypnotics generally have no analgesic action.

3.207   Nitrazepam:

            A.   is chemically similar to chlordiazepoxide

            B.   in therapeutic doses, causes less reduction in REM sleep than other classes of hypnotics

            C.   has a high therapeutic index

            D.   induces hepatic microsomal enzymes if taken for more than one week

            E.   is less liable to induce tolerance and dependence than the barbiturates.

3.208   A.   About 5% of the population have one or more epileptic manifestations at some stage during their lives.

            B.   Birth injury to the brain is one of the major causes of epilepsy.

            C.   Carbamazepine is a benzodiazepine anticonvulsant drug.

            D.   Phenytoin exerts antiepileptic activity without causing marked depression of the central nervous system.

3.209   Anticonvulsant drugs may act by:

            A.   blocking the action of excitatory transmitters

            B.   enhancing the action of inhibitory transmitters

            C.   blocking the release of excitatory transmitters

            D.   enhancing the inactivation of excitatory transmitters

            E.   blocking the inactivation of inhibitory transmitters.

3.210   Both morphine and pethidine induce:

            A.   respiratory depression

            B.   relaxation of the bile duct

            C.   euphoria

            D.   sedation

            E.   nausea and vomiting.

3.211   The therapeutic uses of morphine and related drugs include:

            A.   analgesia

            B.   antidiarrhoeal

            C.   anti-inflammatory

            D.   sedative and relief of anxiety

            E.   cough suppressant.

3.212   Biologically active opioid peptides:

            A.   are all formed from a common precursor prohormone

            B.   have multiple receptors in the central nervous system

            C.   are involved in memory function and pain mechanisms

            D.   are inactivated by peptidase enzymes

            E.   have similar actions to opiate drugs.

3.213   Enkephalins:
    A.   are naturally occurring substances found in the brain and spinal cord
    B.   are nonapeptides
    C.   are involved with the perception of pain
    D.   act at the same receptors as opiates
    E.   are thought to have a presynaptic site of action at the first sensory synapse in nociceptive pathways.

3.214   Met- and leu-enkephalin:
    A.   are pentapeptides
    B.   contain tyrosine and phenylalanine
    C.   differ in structure at one amino acid residue
    D.   act as opiate antagonists on the mouse vas deferens
    E.   are concentrated in the limbic system and the substantia gelatinosa.

3.215   Glycine-mediated synaptic inhibition can be blocked by:
    A.   (+)-tubocurarine
    B.   tetanus toxin
    C.   strychnine
    D.   morphine
    E.   thebaine.

3.216   The binding of [^{3}H]GABA to GABA$_A$ receptors in central nervous tissue can be potentiated by:
    A.   barbiturates
    B.   benzodiazepines
    C.   muscimol
    D.   steroids.

3.217   Picrotoxin:
    A.   is a non-competitive GABA antagonist
    B.   is converted to a more soluble GABA antagonist on N-methylation
    C.   binds to GABA ionophores
    D.   does not significantly inhibit the binding of radiolabelled GABA to rat brain membranes in the absence of chloride ions.

3.218   A.   Most clinically relevant dopamine receptors are in the central nervous system.
    B.   Several effective antipsychotic agents modulate central dopaminergic activity.
    C.   Fluorescence histochemistry can be used to locate dopamine neurones.
    D.   Levodopa therapy used for Parkinson's disease is based on antagonism at dopamine receptors.

3.219   Adenosine:
    A.   inhibits electrically evoked contractions of the guinea pig ileum
    B.   but not ATP, has been shown to depress the activity of many central neurones
    C.   can inhibit the release of several neurotransmitters
    D.   can either stimulate or inhibit adenyl cyclase
    E.   is thought to act on more than one sub-class of receptor.

MCQ

3.220V Induction of anaesthesia:
    i.   is hastened by the use of nitrous oxide
    ii.   is faster if minute respiratory volume is increased
    iii. is faster if the animal is in shock
    iv. is quicker with halothane than with methoxyflurane
    v.   can safely be accomplished using a concentration of oxygen lower than that required for maintenance of anaesthesia.

3.221 Which of the following anaesthetic agents is/are not explosive in the presence of oxygen?
    i.   enflurane
    ii.   methoxyflurane
    iii. halothane
    iv. chloroform
    v.   nitrous oxide.

3.222 Methoxyflurane:
    i.   can be safely administered to a patient with renal failure
    ii.   produces good analgesia
    iii. undergoes little metabolism in the body
    iv. does not depress blood pressure as much as halothane, if anaesthesia is light
    v.   is not a good muscle relaxant.

3.223 Complications of thiopentone administration include:
    i.   laryngospasm
    ii.   hypertension
    iii. respiratory depression
    iv. sensitisation of the heart to adrenaline
    v.   muscle fasciculations.

3.224 Which of the following may be side effects of neuroleptic therapy?
    i.   elevated serum prolactin levels
    ii.   tardive dyskinesia
    iii. malignant hyperpyrexia
    iv. the "on-off" phenomenon
    v.   vomiting.

3.225 In relation to movement disorders and their treatment:
    i.   Self-administration of MPTP has been shown to cause Parkinson's disease.
    ii.   Parkinson's disease is a hyperkinetic, hypertonic syndrome.
    iii. Huntington's disease is a hyperkinetic, hypotonic syndrome.
    iv. Parkinson's disease is a hyperkinetic, hypotonic syndrome.
    v.   Chronic neuroleptic treatment can produce "true" Parkinson's disease.

3.226 Which of the following side effects would be most likely to be a problem after taking levodopa for several years?
    i.   excessive salivation
    ii.   "on-off" effects
    iii. gynaecomastia
    iv. dyskinesia
    v.   tremor.

3.227 Inhibitors of dopa decarboxylase may be given in combination with levodopa to:
    i. increase the ratio of noradrenaline to adrenaline in the basal ganglia
    ii. reduce the incidence of side effects
    iii. facilitate the passage of levodopa across the blood brain barrier
    iv. reduce the formation of dopamine in the periphery.

3.228 Amitriptyline:
    i. is an α-adrenoceptor agonist
    ii. is a neuronal uptake blocker
    iii. potentiates the action of isoprenaline
    iv. has antidepressant properties
    v. potentiates the action of tyramine.

3.229V The combination of etorphine and acepromazine used in animal immobilisation in the wild may be antagonised by:
    i. diprenorphine
    ii. morphine
    iii. naloxone
    iv. methadone.

3.230 Dopamine is an important neurotransmitter in the:
    i. corpus striatum
    ii. nucleus accumbens
    iii. chemoreceptor trigger zone
    iv. raphe nucleus
    v. locus coeruleus.

3.231 Which of the following drugs can cause galactorrhoea?
    i. haloperidol
    ii. levodopa
    iii. chlorpromazine
    iv. tranylcypromine
    v. apomorphine.

3.232 Chlorpromazine is:
    i. a potent dopamine receptor antagonist
    ii. a potent α-adrenoceptor antagonist
    iii. a muscarinic receptor antagonist
    iv. a β-adrenoceptor agonist
    v. a histamine receptor agonist.

ASSERTION / REASON

3.233 Halothane induces anaesthesia very slowly **BECAUSE** halothane has a very low blood:gas solubility coefficient.

3.234 Halothane is seldom used as a general anaesthetic **BECAUSE** halothane has poor analgesic properties.

3.235 The response to a second dose of pentobarbitone 6 hours after a first dose will be decreased **BECAUSE** liver microsomal enzyme activity will be inhibited.

3.236   Diazepam is a better hypnotic than pentobarbitone **BECAUSE** diazepam has a shorter duration of action than pentobarbitone.

3.237   Tyrosine is not useful in the treatment of Parkinson's disease **BECAUSE** tyrosine does not cross the blood brain barrier.

3.238   Bromocriptine is useful in the treatment of Parkinson's disease **BECAUSE** bromocriptine reduces plasma levels of growth hormone in acromegaly.

3.239   In the treatment of Parkinson's disease, bromocriptine produces fewer "end-of-dose" side effects than levodopa **BECAUSE** bromocriptine has a shorter plasma half-life than levodopa.

3.240   Huntington's disease is often characterised by excessive motor movements **BECAUSE** dopamine containing neurones in the substantia nigra degenerate in Huntington's disease.

3.241   Neuroleptics are useful antiemetics **BECAUSE** neuroleptics block dopamine D_2 receptors in the basal ganglia.

3.242   Chlorpromazine and some related phenothiazines are powerful sedative compounds **BECAUSE** chlorpromazine and some related phenothiazines are potent α-adrenoceptor antagonists.

3.243   Haloperidol may produce akathisia **BECAUSE** haloperidol blocks dopamine receptors in the chemoreceptor trigger zone.

3.244   Chlorpromazine is more likely to cause sedation than haloperidol **BECAUSE** chlorpromazine is a more potent antimuscarinic agent then haloperidol.

3.245   Haloperidol may cause postural hypotension **BECAUSE** haloperidol blocks peripheral β-adrenoceptors.

3.246   Carbamazepine is a useful antidepressant drug **BECAUSE** carbamazepine is an effective dopamine receptor antagonist.

3.247   The alkaloid bicuculline is a convulsant **BECAUSE** bicuculline antagonises the action of GABA in the mammalian central nervous system

3.248   Amitriptyline is a useful antidepressant drug **BECAUSE** amitriptyline has antagonist activity at muscarinic receptors.

3.249   Naloxone is used to treat constipation **BECAUSE** naloxone antagonises the action of morphine.

3.250   Apomorphine is a useful emetic in many species **BECAUSE** apomorphine stimulates dopamine receptors in the neostriatum.

3.251   Bromocriptine has been used successfully in the treatment of acromegaly **BECAUSE** the dopamine-mimicking of bromocriptine suppresses prolactin release.

3.252 α-Methyl-p-tyrosine decreases brain levels of dopamine (and noradrenaline) **BECAUSE** α-methyl-p-tyrosine inhibits DOPA decarboxylase.

3.253   Administration of lysergic acid diethylamide results in enhancement of neuronal firing in the lateral geniculate nucleus **BECAUSE** lysergic acid diethylamide antagonises the postsynaptic inhibitory action of 5-hydroxytryptamine at tryptaminergic synapses in the lateral geniculate nucleus.

3.254   Acetylcholine is not involved in central neurotransmission **BECAUSE** acetylcholine does not readily cross the blood brain barrier.

ANSWERS

3.1	F	3.44	F	3.87	T	3.130	B	3.173	A	3.216	C
3.2	F	3.45	T	3.88	T	3.131	C	3.174	B	3.217	B
3.3	F	3.46	T	3.89	T	3.132	A	3.175	C	3.218	D
3.4	F	3.47	T	3.90	T	3.133	B	3.176	D	3.219	B
3.5	F	3.48	T	3.91	F	3.134	C	3.177	C	3.220	E
3.6	F	3.49	T	3.92	T	3.135	C	3.178	A	3.221	E
3.7	T	3.50	F	3.93	F	3.136	C	3.179	B	3.222	C
3.8	T	3.51	F	3.94	F	3.137	A	3.180	D	3.223	B
3.9	T	3.52	F	3.95	F	3.138	C	3.181	B	3.224	A
3.10	F	3.53	F	3.96	T	3.139	E	3.182	E	3.225	B
3.11	T	3.54	F	3.97	T	3.140	C	3.183	A	3.226	C
3.12	T	3.55	F	3.98	F	3.141	C	3.184	A	3.227	C
3.13	F	3.56	T	3.99	F	3.142	E	3.185	D	3.228	C
3.14	T	3.57	T	3.100	F	3.143	E	3.186	B	3.229	B
3.15	T	3.58	T	3.101	T	3.144	B	3.187	B	3.230	A
3.16	F	3.59	F	3.102	T	3.145	B	3.188	E	3.231	B
3.17	T	3.60	F	3.103	F	3.146	C	3.189	C	2.232	A
3.18	T	3.61	F	3.104	T	3.147	C	3.190	B	2.233	E
3.19	T	3.62	F	3.105	F	3.148	D	3.191	A	2.234	D
3.20	T	3.63	F	3.106	T	3.149	D	3.192	D	2.235	C
3.21	F	3.64	T	3.107	F	3.150	A	3.193	D	2.236	E
3.22	T	3.65	F	3.108	T	3.151	C	3.194	C	2.237	C
3.23	T	3.66	F	3.109	F	3.152	C	3.195	B	2.238	B
3.24	T	3.67	F	3.110	F	3.153	A	3.196	D	2.239	C
3.25	F	3.68	F	3.111	T	3.154	D	3.197	A	2.240	C
3.26	F	3.69	F	3.112	T	3.155	B	3.198	D	2.241	B
3.27	F	3.70	F	3.113	F	3.156	C	3.199	B	2.242	A
3.28	F	3.71	T	3.114	F	3.157	C	3.200	E	2.243	B
3.29	T	3.72	F	3.115	F	3.158	C	3.201	D	2.244	B
3.30	T	3.73	F	3.116	T	3.159	D	3.202	E	2.245	C
3.31	T	3.74	F	3.117	T	3.160	C	3.203	E	2.246	E
3.32	T	3.75	T	3.118	T	3.161	C	3.204	C	2.247	A
3.33	F	3.76	F	3.119	T	3.162	C	3.205	C	2.248	B
3.34	F	3.77	T	3.120	F	3.163	A	3.206	B	2.249	D
3.35	T	3.78	T	3.121	T	3.164	D	3.207	D	2.250	B
3.36	T	3.79	F	3.122	T	3.165	E	3.208	C	2.251	B
3.37	F	3.80	F	3.123	F	3.166	B	3.209	D	2.252	C
3.38	T	3.81	T	3.124	T	3.167	C	3.210	B	2.253	C
3.39	F	3.82	T	3.125	F	3.168	A	3.211	C	2.254	D
3.40	T	3.83	T	3.126	F	3.169	A	3.212	A		
3.41	F	3.84	T	3.127	T	3.170	C	3.213	B		
3.42	F	3.85	T	3.128	A	3.171	C	3.214	D		
3.43	F	3.86	F	3.129	B	3.172	A	3.215	A		

4 Autonomic Nervous System

TRUE / FALSE

4.1   The structure of acetylcholine incorporates a quaternary nitrogen and an ester functional group.

4.2   Acetylcholine is synthesised from acetyl CoA and choline.

4.3   The activity of choline acetyltransferase is inhibited by its end product, acetylcholine.

4.4   The block of neuromuscular transmission caused by botulinum toxin can be reversed by neostigmine.

4.5   Stimulation of muscarinic receptors by acetylcholine can cause sweating and salivation.

4.6   McNeil-A-343 stimulates muscarinic receptors on autonomic ganglia.

4.7   The actions of acetylcholine involved in salivary secretion are highly sensitive to blockade by atropine.

4.8   Gallamine is a skeletal neuromuscular blocking agent which selectively stimulates cardiac muscarinic receptors.

4.9   The mechanism for the rapid inactivation of neuronally released acetylcholine is its uptake by a high affinity uptake mechanism.

4.10   Acetylcholinesterase hydrolyses acetylcholine to produce choline and acetyl CoA.

4.11   The hydrolysis of acetylcholine by acetylcholinesterase provides a source of re-usable choline.

4.12   In general, a higher potency of an organophosphorus anticholinesterase as an insecticide is associated with a higher selectivity between insects and man.

4.13   In cases of poisoning by the organophosphorus anticholinesterases, the efficacy of atropine is due to its ability to cleave the covalent bond formed between the enzyme and the inhibitor.

4.14   Neostigmine is an inhibitor of acetylcholinesterase which does not directly stimulate cholinergic receptors.

4.15   Carbamate insecticides and fungicides cause inactivation of acetylcholinesterase which can be reversed by pralidoxime.

4.16   Reversal of suxamethonium-induced neuromuscular blockade is easily achieved by the administration of anticholinesterases.

4.17   Nicotine acts at muscarinic receptors in the smooth muscle membrane.

4.18   Pempidine inhibits the cardiovascular actions of nicotine.

4.19   Tyrosine hydroxylase may be directly inhibited by noradrenaline.

4.20   Noradrenaline-releasing nerve terminals contain the enzyme dopamine β-hydroxylase.

4.21   The rise in blood pressure following i.v. injection of noradrenaline induces a reflex tachycardia.

4.22   Stimulation of α_2-adrenoceptors on adrenergic nerve terminals reduces transmitter output.

4.23   Clonidine stimulates α_2-adrenoceptors.

4.24   Selective β_1-adrenoceptor agonists are beneficial in the treatment of bronchospasm.

4.25   Terbutaline is a selective stimulant of myocardial β-adrenoceptors.

4.26   Dobutamine and isoprenaline, in equiactive inotropic doses, have comparable chronotropic effects.

4.27   Non-selective α-adrenoceptor antagonists increase neural release of noradrenaline.

4.28   α-Adrenoceptor antagonists may be useful in the treatment of chilblains.

4.29   Yohimbine is a selective inhibitor of α_1-adrenoceptors.

4.30   Phenoxybenzamine is a selective α_2-adrenoceptor antagonist.

4.31   Prazosin preferentially blocks α_2-adrenoceptors.

4.32   Therapeutic doses of cardioselective β-adrenoceptor antagonists only affect myocardial β-adrenoceptors.

4.33   β-Adrenoceptor blocking drugs lower cardiac output.

4.34   Renin release from the kidney can be blocked by propranolol.

4.35   Propranolol is safe to use in patients with a history of bronchospasm.

4.36   Monoamine oxidase inhibitors have both antihypertensive and antidepressant activity.

4.37   The major problem associated with the clinical use of monoamine oxidase inhibitors is postural hypotension.

4.38   α-Methyldopa is metabolised to α-methylnoradrenaline in the sympathetic nerve terminals.

4.39 Rauwolfia alkaloids may cause symptoms of excessive parasympathetic activity including bradycardia, salivation and diarrhoea.

4.40 There is no effective antagonist of the effects of depolarising blocking drugs at the skeletal neuromuscular junction.

4.41 Suxamethonium acts like an excess of acetylcholine.

4.42 Atracurium is the shortest acting of the non-depolarising muscle relaxants.

CORRECT OPTION

4.43 Which of the following criteria is not necessary for a substance to be considered as a neurotransmitter?
    A.   It is presynaptically localised in specific neurones.
    B.   It is released in effective concentrations by physiological stimuli.
    C.   The substance demonstrates identity of postsynaptic action at the synapse under investigation
    D.   Its action is antagonised by therapeutically useful drugs.
    E.   Mechanisms exist at the synapse that will terminate its action.

4.44 Indicate the non-conforming pair of drugs:
    A.   propranolol   isoprenaline
    B.   atropine   muscarine
    C.   phenoxybenzamine   tolazoline
    D.   phentolamine   noradrenaline
    E.   pentolinium   nicotine.

4.45 Indicate the non-conforming pair of drugs:
    A.   noradrenaline   pilocarpine
    B.   adrenaline   isoprenaline
    C.   physostigmine   neostigmine
    D.   muscarine   methacholine
    E.   acetylcholine   carbachol.

4.46 Indicate the the non-conforming pair of drugs:
    A. muscarine   atropine
    B. noradrenaline   suxamethonium
    C. isoprenaline   propranolol
    D. acetylcholine   hexamethonium
    E. nicotine   (+)-tubocurarine.

4.47 Indicate the non-conforming drug:
    A.   muscarine
    B.   acetylcholine
    C.   methacholine
    D.   hyoscine
    E.   carbachol.

4.48   Indicate the non-conforming drug:
    A.   phentolamine
    B.   atropine
    C.   pilocarpine
    D.   muscarine
    E.   methacholine.

4.49   Which of the following drugs does not exert its action by inhibition of enzymatic breakdown of transmitter?
    A.   di-isopropyl phosphorofluoridate (DFP)
    B.   pargyline
    C.   tranylcypromine
    D.   physostigmine
    E.   botulinum toxin.

4.50   Mimicking the action of the transmitter at the postsynaptic receptor site is the action of all of the following drugs except:
    A.   reserpine
    B.   isoprenaline
    C.   nicotine
    D.   methacholine
    E.   phenylephrine.

4.51   Myasthenia gravis is a disease characterised by:
    A.   blockade of excitation-secretion coupling in the presynaptic terminal
    B.   a reduction in the number of acetylcholine receptors available at the end-plate
    C.   the spread of acetylcholine receptors to non-end-plate regions of muscle fibres
    D.   demyelination of motor axons.

4.52   Which one of the following drugs can directly inhibit acetylcholine release?
    A.   α-methyl-p-tyrosine
    B.   botulinum toxin
    C.   arecoline
    D.   GABA
    E.   hemicholinium.

4.53   Botulinum toxin:
    A.   abolishes action potentials in peripheral nerves
    B.   only affects primates
    C.   blocks the spontaneous and evoked release of acetylcholine at the neuromuscular junction
    D.   is a phospholipase.

4.54   Which of the following effects would not be expected from a dose of carbachol?
    A.   reduction in heart rate
    B.   reduction in intraocular pressure
    C.   miosis
    D.   diarrhoea
    E.   urinary retention.

4.55   In the eye, atropine lengthens the near point by:
        A.   blocking parasympathetic innervation of the circular muscle of
             the iris
        B.   blocking parasympathetic innervation of the radial muscle of the
             iris
        C.   blocking parasympathetic innervation of the ciliary muscle
        D.   stimulating the central nervous system
        E.   all of the above.

4.56   Which of the following plants does not contain hyoscine?
        A.   *Atropa belladonna*
        B.   *Hyoscyamus niger*
        C.   *Datura stramonium*
        D.   *Strychnos nux-vomica*.

4.57   Which of the following muscarinic responses is inhibited most effectively
        by pirenzepine?
        A.   secretion of gastric acid
        B.   contraction of the smooth muscle of the gut
        C.   contraction of the smooth muscle of the bladder
        D.   contraction of the circular muscle of the eye
        E.   secretion from sweat glands.

4.58   Which of the following anticholinesterases does not have a reversible
        effect?
        A.   di-isopropylphosphofluoridate
        B.   neostigmine
        C.   edrophonium
        D.   ambenonium
        E.   physostigmine.

4.59   Which of the following would not normally be an indication for the use of
        anticholinesterase agents?
        A.   myasthenia gravis
        B.   glaucoma
        C.   atony of the smooth muscle of the gastrointestinal tract
        D.   constipation
        E.   atropine intoxication.

4.60   The toxic effects of carbamate anticholinesterase insecticides are best
        treated by:
        A.   atropine
        B.   pralidoxime
        C.   atropine and pralidoxime
        D.   none of the above.

4.61   (+)-Tubocurarine blocks the neuromuscular action of acetylcholine by:
        A.   blocking its synthesis
        B.   blocking its release
        C.   breaking it down in the synapse
        D.   reversibly blocking its receptor sites
        E.   reversibly binding to acetylcholine molecules.

4.62   Neostigmine:
        A.   blocks acetylcholine receptors
        B.   depolarises the end-plate regions of muscle cells
        C.   reverses the blockade produced by suxamethonium
        D.   reverses the blockade produced by (+)-tubocurarine
        E.   potentiates muscarinic but not nicotinic responses to
             acetylcholine.

4.63   Which of the following applies to both (+)-tubocurarine and
        suxamethonium?
        A.   causes muscle fasciculations when injected rapidly
        B.   is a naturally occurring compound
        C.   ether anaesthesia increases the degree of neuromuscular block
        D.   causes respiratory paralysis by a peripheral mechanism
        E.   the effect can be overcome by the administration of neostigmine.

4.64   Which of the following non-depolarising muscle relaxants has the
        shortest duration of action?
        A.   (+)-tubocurarine
        B.   gallamine
        C.   alcuronium
        D.   pancuronium
        E.   atracurium.

4.65   Which of the following agents interacts with nicotinic receptors?
        A.   lobeline
        B.   muscarine
        C.   strychnine
        D.   LSD.

4.66-4.68

4.66   atropine

4.67   neostigmine

4.68   carbachol

        For each of the drugs listed above, indicate whether it:

        A.   is used in pre-operative medication
        B.   is used in the treatment of myasthenia gravis
        C.   irreversibly inhibits acetylcholinesterase
        D.   has both nicotinic and muscarinic agonist activity
        E.   has predominantly muscarinic agonist activity.

4.69   Which of the following sequences correctly describes the synthesis of
        noradrenaline?
        A.   tyrosine - dobutamine - dopa - noradrenaline
        B.   phenylalanine - tyrosine - dopamine - dopa - noradrenaline
        C.   tyrosine - phenylalanine - dopa - dopamine - noradrenaline
        D.   phenylalanine - tyrosine - dopa - dopamine - noradrenaline
        E.   phenylalanine - tyrosine - dopa - dopamine - adrenaline -
             noradrenaline.

4.70   Which of the following conversions is the rate-limiting step in the synthesis of noradrenaline?
    A.   dopamine to noradrenaline
    B.   dopa to dopamine
    C.   adrenaline to noradrenaline
    D.   phenylalanine to tyrosine
    E.   tyrosine to dopa.

4.71   The most important mechanism for the inactivation of noradrenaline is:
    A.   metabolism by acetylcholinesterase
    B.   metabolism by catechol-O-methyltransferase
    C.   metabolism by monoamine oxidase
    D.   uptake into smooth muscle
    E.   uptake into sympathetic nerve terminals.

4.72   Which of the following effects would not generally occur after activation of the sympathetic nervous system?
    A.   mydriasis
    B.   decrease in conduction velocity in the atria
    C.   ejaculation
    D.   decrease in gastric motility
    E.   tachycardia.

4.73   The cardiovascular actions of methoxamine can be blocked by:
    A.   propranolol
    B.   phentolamine
    C.   amitriptyline
    D.   pargyline
    E.   nicotine.

4.74   Which of the following effects of adrenaline is mediated by stimulation of α-adrenoceptors?
    A.   tachycardia
    B.   relaxation of bronchiolar smooth muscle
    C.   increased blood flow through skeletal muscle
    D.   release of renin from the kidney
    E.   vasoconstriction of the splanchnic vessels.

4.75   An affinity for β-adrenoceptors is manifested by all of the following except:
    A.   noradrenaline
    B.   propranolol
    C.   isoprenaline
    D.   phentolamine
    E.   salbutamol.

4.76   Which of the following does not have agonist activity at β-adrenoceptors in respiratory smooth muscle?
    A.   adrenaline
    B.   isoprenaline
    C.   terbutaline
    D.   propranolol
    E.   salbutamol.

4.77 Isoprenaline exerts its cardiovascular actions at:
  A.   α-adrenoceptors only
  B. β_1-adrenoceptors only
  C. β_2-adrenoceptors only
  D. β_1- and β_2-adrenoceptors
  E.   α-, β_1- and β_2-adrenoceptors.

4.78 The side effects of isoprenaline when used as a bronchodilator include:
  A.   bradycardia
  B.   gastric irritation
  C.   palpitations
  D.   agranulocytosis
  E.   urinary retention.

4.79 β-Adrenoceptor blocking drugs which are partial agonists:
  A.   stimulate and block β-adrenoceptors
  B.   stimulate β_2- and block β_1-adrenoceptors
  C.   stimulate α-adrenoceptors before blocking β-adrenoceptors
  D.   are the treatment of choice for tachyarrhythmias
  E.   reduce heart rate because of stimulation of presynaptic β-adrenoceptors.

4.80 In patients being treated with anti-diabetic drugs, β-adrenoceptor antagonists must be used with caution because they:
  A.   enhance growth hormone secretion
  B.   suppress endogenous catecholamine-induced glycogenolysis
  C.   enhance endogenous catecholamine-induced glycogenolysis
  D.   suppress the cardiovascular symptoms of hypoglycaemia
  E.   antagonise the effects of biguanide-induced hyperglycaemia.

4.81 Which of the following β-adrenoceptor antagonists exhibits intrinsic sympathomimetic activity?
  A.   propranolol
  B.   pindolol
  C.   labetolol.

4.82 In thyrotoxicosis, propranolol:
  A.   reduces the increased levels of circulating catecholamines
  B.   blocks the stimulating effects of autoantibodies on thyrotrophin receptors
  C.   abolishes the clinical manifestations of sympathetic overactivity
  D.   restores the ratio of thyroxine to tri-iodothyronine in plasma to normal
  E.   none of the above.

4.83 Deprenyl selectively inhibits:
  A.   tyrosine hydroxylase
  B.   monoamine oxidase A
  C.   DOPA decarboxylase
  D.   fructase
  E.   monoamine oxidase B.

4.84   The mechanism of action of pargyline may be best categorised as:
    A.   Uptake$_1$ blockade
    B.   Uptake$_2$ blockade
    C.   monoamine oxidase inhibition
    D.   catechol-O-methyltransferase inhibition
    E.   α-adrenoceptor antagonism.

4.85   Which of the following is not contraindicated in patients taking monoamine oxidase inhibitors?
    A.   beer
    B.   red wine
    C.   red meat
    D.   chicken liver
    E.   cheese.

4.86   Which of the following drugs does not lower blood pressure?
    A.   reserpine
    B.   tolazoline
    C.   guanethidine
    D.   salbutamol
    E.   tyramine.

4.87   Which of the following drugs does not lower blood pressure?
    A.   prazosin
    B.   phenoxybenzamine
    C.   phenylephrine
    D.   pargyline
    E.   propranolol.

4.88-4.94

4.88   blocks the release of noradrenaline from the adrenergic neurone

4.89   stimulates β$_2$-adrenoceptors

4.90   mimics the inotropic stimulant actions of noradrenaline

4.91   blocks the β$_1$-adrenoceptor-mediated effects of noradrenaline

4.92   blocks the α-adrenoceptor-mediated effects of noradrenaline

4.93   is taken up into the adrenergic nerve terminal

4.94   is used in the treatment of cardiac arrhythmias

For each of the statements above, indicate whether it applies to:

    A.   dobutamine
    B.   salbutamol
    C.   metoprolol
    D.   guanethidine
    E.   phentolamine.

4.95-4.97

4.95   salbutamol

4.96   tyramine

4.97   methoxamine

For each of the drugs above, indicate whether it is:

A.   a non-specific smooth muscle relaxant
B.   a selective β_2-adrenoceptor agonist
C.   a selective α-adrenoceptor agonist
D.   a monoamine oxidase inhibitor
E.   an indirectly acting pressor agent.

4.98-4.100

4.98   tyramine

4.99   propranolol

4.100   amitriptyline

For each of the drugs above, indicate whether it:

A.   inhibits uptake of noradrenaline into nerve terminals
B.   competitively inhibits the actions of noradrenaline at
       β-adrenoceptors
C.   depletes the stores of noradrenaline
D.   blocks the release of transmitter from the adrenergic nerve
       terminal
E.   causes the release of transmitter from the adrenergic nerve
       terminal.

4.101-4.103

4.101   reserpine

4.102   butoxamine

4.103 α-methyl-p-tyrosine

For each of the drugs above, indicated whether its action is best described
by:

A.   dopamine granule depletion
B.   tyrosine hydroxylase inhibition
C.   selective β_2-adrenoceptor blockade
D.   neurone blockade
E.   increased release of dopamine into the synapse.

4.104 Indicate the non-conforming drug:
  A.   salbutamol
  B.   isoprenaline
  C.   propranolol
  D.   terbutaline
  E.   orciprenaline.

4.105 Suxamethonium is:
  A.   a competitive antagonist at nicotinic receptors
  B.   a competitive antagonist at muscarinic receptors
  C.   a non-competitive antagonist at nicotinic receptors
  D.   a non-competitive antagonist at muscarinic receptors
  E.   an inhibitor of acetylcholine release.

INCORRECT OPTION

4.106
  A.   Acetylcholine binds to nicotinic receptors.
  B.   Lignocaine blocks sodium channels.
  C.   Suxamethonium binds to nicotinic receptors.
  D.   Neostigmine binds to acetylcholinesterase.
  E.   Mepyramine binds to nicotinic receptors.

4.107 Acetylcholine is a neurotransmitter:
  A.   at skeletal neuromuscular junctions, where it is antagonised by (+)-tubocurarine
  B.   at all autonomic ganglia, where it is antagonised by hexamethonium
  C.   at postganglionic parasympathetic nerves, where it is antagonised by muscarine
  D.   which is synthesised by choline acetyltransferase
  E.   which is hydrolysed by acetylcholinesterase.

4.108 Botulinum toxin:
  A.   is a single chain polypeptide when released
  B.   mimics the effects of denervation at the neuromuscular junction
  C.   causes the disappearance of vesicles from cholinergic terminals
  D.   must be taken into nerve terminals to produce its effects
  E.   undergoes two proteolytic reactions to become fully active.

4.109 The actions of carbachol include:
  A.   reduction in heart rate
  B.   inhibition of secretions in the respiratory tract
  C.   vasodilation
  D.   increased gastrointestinal motility
  E.   constriction of the pupil.

4.110 Antimuscarinic drugs are useful in:
  A.   glaucoma
  B.   Parkinson's disease
  C.   pre-anaesthetic medication
  D.   treatment of poisoning with anticholinesterases
  E.   symptomatic treatment of the common cold.

4.111   The actions of hyoscine include:
    A.   prevention of motion sickness
    B.   pupillary dilation
    C.   convulsions
    D.   reduced gastrointestinal motility
    E.   reduced bronchial secretions.

4.112   The anticholinesterase agents:
    A.   can be divided into reversible and irreversible types
    B.   include neostigmine and physostigmine
    C.   can produce miosis and lacrimation
    D.   are useful as bronchodilators
    E.   may be useful in the treatment of myasthenia gravis.

4.113   Acetylcholinesterase:
    A.   inactivates atropine by hydrolysis
    B.   is reversibly inhibited by neostigmine
    C.   hydrolyses a carbamate group more slowly than an acetyl group
    D.   is irreversibly inhibited by di-isopropyl phosphorofluoridate
    E.   inhibition can lead to increased tissue levels of acetylcholine.

4.114   Ganglion blocking drugs:
    A.   decrease gastrointestinal motility
    B.   decrease bronchial and salivary secretions
    C.   produce postural hypotension
    D.   may cause urine retention
    E.   inhibit the actions of acetylcholine at muscarinic receptor sites.

4.115   Noradrenaline is inactivated by:
    A.   specific neuronal uptake
    B.   dopamine β-hydroxylase
    C.   catechol-O-methyltransferase
    D.   monoamine oxidase.

4.116   Adrenaline causes:
    A.   bronchodilation by stimulating β_2-adrenoceptors
    B.   tachycardia by stimulating β_1-adrenoceptors
    C.   vasodilation by stimulating β_1-adrenoceptors
    D.   vasoconstriction by stimulating α-adrenoceptors
    E.   increased cardiac contractility by stimulating β_1-adrenoceptors.

4.117   A.   Salbutamol is a selective β_1-adrenoceptor stimulant.
    B.   Foetal tachycardia can result from using salbutamol.
    C.   Infusion of salbutamol can lower blood pressure.
    D.   Salbutamol is used to delay parturition.
    E.   Salbutamol is used in the treatment of asthma.

4.118 β-Adrenoceptor blocking drugs may:
    A.   precipitate heart failure
    B.   aggravate symptoms of peripheral vascular disease
    C.   precipitate asthma
    D.   increase maximal exercise performance in healthy individuals
    E.   increase plasma lipids.

4.119   Propranolol:
          A.   has an antagonist actions at β_1- and β_2-adrenoceptors
          B.   reduces post-exercise heart rate
          C.   may reduce resting heart rate
          D.   may alter insulin requirements of diabetic patients
          E.   causes bronchodilation *via* β_2-adrenoceptors.

4.120   Among the actions of propranolol which are due to β_1-adrenoceptor
        blockade are:
          A.   decrease in heart rate
          B.   prolongation of A-V conduction time
          C.   reduction in cardiac contractility
          D.   reduced peripheral blood flow
          E.   antagonism of the cardiac actions of catecholamines.

4.121 β-Adrenoceptor blocking drugs may produce the following effects:
          A.   severe asthma
          B.   skeletal muscle tremor
          C.   bradycardia
          D.   cardiac failure
          E.   dreams and nightmares.

4.122   Propranolol blocks the vasodepressor effects of:
          A.   isoprenaline
          B.   adrenaline
          C.   histamine
          D.   salbutamol
          E.   terbutaline.

MCQ

4.123   Cholinergic stimulation of the:
          i.   sphincter muscle of the iris produces miosis
          ii.   SA node of the heart causes bradycardia
          iii. adrenal medulla causes secretion of adrenaline and
                noradrenaline
          iv.   male sex organs causes ejaculation
          v.   atria of the heart causes an increase in contractility.

4.124   Which of the following symptoms might be evident in a case of atropine
        overdosage?
          i.   blurred vision
          ii.   difficulty in micturition
          iii. dilated pupils
          iv.   diarrhoea
          v.   bradycardia.

4.125   Symptoms of poisoning by organophosphorus insecticides include:
          i.   pupil constriction
          ii.   bradycardia
          iii. vomiting and diarrhoea
          iv.   salivation
          v.   bronchoconstriction.

4.126   Intravenous administration of neostigmine causes:
      i.   bradycardia
      ii.   excessive secretions
      iii.   bronchoconstriction
      iv.   contraction of the gut.

4.127   Which of the following drugs has/have potent agonist activity at muscarinic and nicotinic receptors and is/are insensitive to acetylcholinesterase?
      i.   arecoline
      ii.   acetylcholine
      iii.   carbachol
      iv.   methacholine
      v.   bethanechol.

4.128   Which of the following muscle relaxants is/are competitive blocking agent/s at the motor end-plate?
      i.   pancuronium bromide
      ii.   (+)-tubocurarine
      iii.   alcuronium
      iv.   decamethonium bromide
      v.   suxamethonium chloride.

4.129   Noradrenaline is a neurotransmitter:
      i.   which stimulates both muscarinic and nicotinic receptors
      ii.   at postganglionic sympathetic nerves
      iii.   which is inactivated by dopamine b-hydroxylase
      iv.   which is released in response to stress
      v.   which is involved in energy conservation processes.

4.130   Adrenaline is used in the emergency treatment of anaphylaxis because it:
      i.   stimulates cardiac β_1-adrenoceptors
      ii.   blocks α-adrenoceptors in the peripheral arterioles
      iii.   stimulates pulmonary β_2-adrenoceptors
      iv.   reduces oxygen delivery to the skeletal muscle
      v.   blocks prostaglandin release in the kidney.

4.131   Prazosin:
      i.   selectively blocks α_1-adrenoceptors
      ii.   has an enhanced effect in the presence of salt depletion
      iii.   affects human arteries and veins in widely different concentrations
      iv.   in high concentrations inhibits phosphodiesterases
      v.   is associated with severe postural hypotension in elderly patients.

4.132   Blockade of postsynaptic α-adrenoceptors causes:
      i.   hypotension
      ii.   bradycardia
      iii.   nasal stuffiness
      iv.   reduced gastrointestinal motility
      v.   mydriasis.

4.133 β-Adrenoceptor blocking drugs may adversely affect patients with:
      i.   a history of asthma
      ii.   diabetes mellitus
      iii.   congestive cardiac failure
      iv.   thyrotoxicosis
      v.   idiopathic hypertropic subaortic stenosis (IHSS).

4.134 Amitriptyline:
    i.   does not affect monoamine oxidase
    ii.   is a neuronal uptake blocker
    iii. has antidepressant properties
    iv. potentiates the actions of isoprenaline
    v.   potentiates the actions of tyramine.

ASSERTION / REASON

4.135 Hemicholinium enhances the synthesis of acetylcholine **BECAUSE** hemicholinium increases levels of choline in the nerve terminal.

4.136 The venom of the black widow spider can, on occasions, be lethal **BECAUSE** the venom of the black widow spider blocks Ca^{2+}-induced exocytosis of acetylcholine.

4.137 Tropicamide is used in preference to atropine for ophthalmic examination **BECAUSE** atropine dose not produce sufficient dilation of the pupil.

4.138 Anticholinergic drugs are bronchodilators **BECAUSE** stimulation of the vagus nerve causes relaxation of airway smooth muscle.

4.139 Neostigmine causes a marked increase in the cholinergic activity of carbachol **BECAUSE** neostigmine inhibits the degradation of carbachol.

4.140 Atropine and neostigmine must never be administered together **BECAUSE** neostigmine has a much shorter duration of action than atropine.

4.141 Physostigmine is useful in the treatment of glaucoma **BECAUSE** physostigmine is an irreversible anticholinesterase.

4.142 Guanethidine lowers blood pressure **BECAUSE** guanethidine is a selective α_1-adrenoceptor antagonist.

4.143 Subcutaneous injection of adrenaline is used in the treatment of anaphylaxis **BECAUSE** adrenaline is released from the adrenal medulla in the physiological response to stress.

4.144 Isoprenaline decreases both blood pressure and heart rate **BECAUSE** isoprenaline stimulates both β_1- and β_2-adrenoceptors.

4.145 Prazosin increases blood pressure **BECAUSE** prazosin is a selective α_1-adrenoceptor antagonist.

4.146 Stimulation of prejunctional α-adrenoceptors leads to vasoconstriction **BECAUSE** prejunctional α-adrenoceptors are predominantly of the α_2-subtype.

4.147 β-Adrenoceptor blocking drugs may aggravate symptoms of peripheral vascular disease **BECAUSE** β-adrenoceptor blocking drugs may precipitate asthmatic attacks.

4.148 Monoamine oxidase inhibitors are contraindicated in hypertension **BECAUSE** the accumulation of noradrenaline in the central nervous system which occurs with monoamine oxidase inhibition causes an increase in systemic blood pressure.

4.149 (+)-Tubocurarine is a competitive blocker of the action of acetylcholine at the skeletal neuroeffector junction **BECAUSE** (+)-tubocurarine transiently stimulates nicotinic receptors causing depolarisation of the muscle membrane.

ANSWERS

4.1	T	4.26	F	4.51	B	4.76	D	4.101	A	4.126	E
4.2	T	4.27	T	4.52	B	4.77	D	4.102	C	4.127	B
4.3	F	4.28	T	4.53	C	4.78	C	4.103	B	4.128	A
4.4	F	4.29	F	4.54	E	4.79	A	4.104	C	4.129	C
4.5	T	4.30	F	4.55	C	4.80	B	4.105	C	4.130	B
4.6	T	4.31	F	4.56	D	4.81	B	4.106	E	4.131	E
4.7	T	4.32	F	4.57	A	4.82	C	4.107	C	4.132	B
4.8	F	4.33	T	4.58	A	4.83	E	4.108	C	4.133	A
4.9	F	4.34	T	4.59	D	4.84	C	4.109	B	4.134	A
4.10	F	4.35	F	4.60	A	4.85	C	4.110	A	4.135	E
4.11	T	4.36	T	4.61	D	4.86	E	4.111	C	4.136	C
4.12	F	4.37	F	4.62	D	4.87	C	4.112	D	4.137	C
4.13	F	4.38	T	4.63	D	4.88	D	4.113	A	4.138	C
4.14	T	4.39	T	4.64	E	4.89	B	4.114	E	4.139	E
4.15	F	4.40	T	4.65	A	4.90	A	4.115	B	4.140	D
4.16	F	4.41	T	4.66	A	4.91	C	4.116	C	4.141	C
4.17	F	4.42	T	4.67	B	4.92	E	4.117	A	4.142	C
4.18	T	4.43	D	4.68	D	4.93	D	4.118	D	4.143	B
4.19	T	4.44	C	4.69	D	4.94	C	4.119	E	4.144	D
4.20	T	4.45	A	4.70	E	4.95	B	4.120	D	4.145	D
4.21	F	4.46	B	4.71	E	4.96	E	4.121	B	4.146	D
4.22	T	4.47	D	4.72	B	4.97	C	4.122	C	4.147	B
4.23	T	4.48	A	4.73	B	4.98	E	4.123	A	4.148	E
4.24	F	4.49	E	4.74	E	4.99	B	4.124	A	4.149	C
4.25	F	4.50	A	4.75	D	4.100	A	4.125	E		

5 Local Anaesthetics

TRUE / FALSE

5.1   The order in which sensation is lost following infiltration of a local anaesthetic is pain, then temperature, then touch.

5.2   Myelinated nerve fibres and unmyelinated nerve fibres are equally susceptible to the action of local anaesthetics.

5.3   Epidural anaesthesia affects only the ventral nerve roots leaving the spinal cord.

5.4   Clinically useful local anaesthetics are almost all weak bases.

5.5   At physiological pH, the majority of local anaesthetic molecules exist in the cationic form.

5.6   The ideal pK_a for a local anaesthetic is such that 50% of the drug exists as free base at physiological pH.

5.7   Lignocaine solutions containing adrenaline should not be used for digital nerve blocks.

5.8   Hypersensitivity is more likely with a local anaesthetic of the ester class than with one of the amide class.

CORRECT OPTION

5.9   The mechanism of action of local anaesthetics involves:
        A.   antagonism of Mg^{2+} receptors on cell membranes
        B.   prevention of transcription of RNA
        C.   competition for Ca^{2+} receptors which control Na^+ permeability
        D.   prevention of acetylcholine release at synapses
        E.   inactivation of nociceptors on sensory nerve terminals.

5.10 - 5.14

5.10   amylocaine

5.11   benzocaine

5.12   lignocaine

5.13   bupivicaine

5.14   cocaine

For each of the drugs listed above, indicate whether it is:

A.   a benzoic acid ester
B.   a para-amino benzoic acid ester
C.   a meta-amino benzoic acid ester
D.   an amide
E.   an azide.

5.15   Lignocaine, when given intradermally as a local anaesthetic, has a longer
duration of action than procaine because it:
A.   has a higher pK_a and thus more deeply penetrates the nerve fibres

B.   is a secondary amine which irreversibly depolarises afferent nerve
fibres
C.   has vasoconstrictor activity, thereby reducing systemic absorption
D.   is an amide derivative which is resistant to hydrolysis by plasma
esterases
E.   none of the above.

5.16   Which of the following local anaesthetics is not effective on topical
administration?
A.   lignocaine
B.   procaine
C.   prilocaine
D.   cinchocaine
E.   cocaine.

INCORRECT OPTION

5.17   Lignocaine:
A.   is absorbed from mucous membranes
B.   is useful in the treatment of cardiac arrhythmias
C.   has a longer duration of action than procaine
D.   has anticonvulsant activity
E.   is metabolised in the liver.

5.18   In excitable tissues, local anaesthetics:
    A.   prevent the transient increase in cell membrane permeability to Na^+ which occurs when the membrane is depolarised
    B.   decrease the resting cell membrane permeability to Na^+
    C.   decrease the resting cell membrane permeability to K^+
    D.   produce hyperpolarisation of the cell membrane as a consequence of changes in cell membrane permeability
    E.   may compete with Ca^{2+} at an intracellular site which controls membrane permeability.

MCQ

5.19   Epidural anaesthesia may be preferred to spinal anaesthesia because:
    i.   there is less risk of infection of cerebrospinal fluid (CSF)
    ii.   motor nerve roots are unaffected
    iii.   there is less risk of persistent CSF leak
    iv.   smaller amounts of local anaesthetic are required
    v.   the technique is less difficult.

5.20   Local anaesthetics produce nerve conduction block:
    i.   by irreversible damage to the myelin sheath
    ii.   only in sensory nerves
    iii.   by inhibiting mitochondrial respiration
    iv.   by decreasing permeability of neurones to Na^+
    v.   by decreasing the activity of fast Na^+ channels.

5.21   Local anaesthetics:
    i.   are active in the cationic form
    ii.   suppress nerve conduction by reducing the passage of Na^+ across the cell membrane during depolarisation
    iii.   in high doses may prolong the PR interval in the electrocardiogram
    iv.   only affect the transmission of action potentials in peripheral nerves
    v.   exhibit tachyphylaxis with repeated injections.

ASSERTION / REASON

5.22   Local anaesthetics with an amide group have a short duration of action **BECAUSE** local anaesthetics with an amide group are metabolised by the liver.

5.23   Adrenaline prolongs the duration of local anaesthetics **BECAUSE** adrenaline inhibits plasma cholinesterases.

5.24   Local anaesthetics are less effective in the presence of pus **BECAUSE** the acidic environment reduces the concentration of pharmacologically active cations.

5.25 Amethocaine is a useful corneal surface local anaesthetic **BECAUSE** amethocaine has a duration of action of about 20 minutes.

5.26 Prilocaine is never combined with a vasoconstrictor **BECAUSE** prilocaine has intrinsic vasoconstrictor properties.

5.27 Lignocaine must not be administered parenterally **BECAUSE** lignocaine is metabolised to monoethylglycine and xylidine.

5.28 Lignocaine has a short duration of action as a local anaesthetic **BECAUSE** lignocaine is a rapidly hydrolysed by tissue pseudocholinesterase.

ANSWERS

5.1	T	5.7	T	5.13	D	5.19	B	5.25	C
5.2	F	5.8	T	5.14	A	5.20	D	5.26	D
5.3	F	5.9	C	5.15	D	5.21	A	5.27	D
5.4	T	5.10	A	5.16	B	5.22	D	5.28	E
5.5	T	5.11	B	5.17	D	5.23	C		
5.6	F	5.12	D	5.18	D	5.24	C		

6 Non-narcotic Analgesics, Autacoids

TRUE / FALSE

6.1   Agents which decrease cyclic AMP levels in mast cells inhibit the release of histamine and other autacoids.

Both histamine and 5-hydroxytryptamine:

6.2   are synthesised from an amino acid and excreted as a carboxylic acid.

6.3   are antagonised by cyproheptadine.

Elevated 3',5'-cyclic AMP in respiratory tissue mast cells may result from treatment with:

6.4   acetylcholine.

6.5   prostaglandin $F_{2\alpha}$

6.6   salbutamol.

6.7   adrenaline.

6.8   Histamine is synthesised by the decarboxylation of histidine.

6.9   Activation of histamine H_1-receptors causes contraction of bronchial and gastrointestinal smooth muscle.

6.10   In the triple response following intradermal injection of histamine, the wheal is due to increased microvascular permeability.

Histamine H_1 -receptor antagonists:

6.11   are the treatment of choice for acute anaphylactic shock.

6.12   are used to treat peptic ulcer.

6.13   are often mild sedatives.

6.14V   are useful for the treatment of motion sickness in cats and dogs.

6.15   Central nervous system actions are less likely to be produced by histamine H_1-receptor antagonists of the alkylamine class than those of the ethanolamine class.

6.16   The histamine H_2-receptor antagonist cimetidine inhibits both the wheal and flare response following intradermal infiltration of histamine.

6.17   3-Methyl histamine is a selective histamine H_2-receptor agonist.

6.18   The effects of bradykinin on microvascular permeability are enhanced by prostaglandin E_2.

6.19   The stimulant action of bradykinin on pain afferent fibres involves the formation and liberation of prostaglandins.

6.20   The nonsteroidal anti-inflammatory drugs all inhibit the enzyme cyclo-oxygenase.

6.21   Aspirin differs from the other nonsteroidal anti-inflammatory drugs because it inhibits the enzyme lipoxygenase.

6.22   Thromboxane A_2 is formed from linoleic acid.

6.23   Thromboxane A_2 is a stable product formed from thromboxane B_2.

6.24   Prostaglandin I_2 degrades to 6-ketoprostaglandin $F_{1\alpha}$.

6.25   Prostacyclin inhibits platelet aggregation.

6.26   Prostaglandin E_2 and prostaglandin I_2 stimulate gastric secretion of pepsin and hydrochloric acid.

6.27   Prostaglandin E_2 and prostaglandin $F_{2\alpha}$ are inactivated during a single passage through the pulmonary circulation.

6.28   Prostaglandin $F_{2\alpha}$ relaxes uterine smooth muscle.

6.29   Prostaglandin $F_{2\alpha}$ is a potent bronchoconstrictor.

6.30   Asthmatic patients are more sensitive than non-asthmatics to inhalation of prostaglandin $F_{2\alpha}$.

6.31   Suppression of the nociceptive actions of kinins by aspirin involves inhibition of prostaglandin formation.

6.32   Salicylic acid conjugates are responsible for the antipyretic action of aspirin.

6.33   Salicylates may displace other nonsteroidal anti-inflammatory agents from their protein binding sites.

6.34   When an overdose of aspirin has been taken, increased urinary excretion of the drug can be achieved by the administration of sodium bicarbonate.

6.35   Aspirin will not lower body temperature unless it is raised above normal.

6.36   In pyrexia due to infections, salicylates act by diminishing body heat production.

6.37   Aspirin exerts its anti-inflammatory effect by inhibiting histidine decarboxylase.

6.38   Acetylsalicylic acid reduces sensitisation of sensory nerve endings caused by tissue injury by inhibiting the synthesis of prostaglandin E_2.

6.39   Small doses of aspirin divert the prostaglandin pathway towards excess production of thromboxane.

6.40   For adequate anti-inflammatory effect, the plasma concentrations of salicylates should be in the range of 1.1-2.2 mmol/l.

6.41   Aspirin is the drug of first choice in the treatment of gout.

6.42   Aspirin and paracetamol are equipotent as anti-inflammatory agents.

6.43   If a patient receiving aspirin for rheumatoid arthritis experiences an exacerbation of asthma, it is likely that the patient will tolerate indomethacin without ill-effect.

6.44   In normal therapeutic doses, paracetamol has more side effects than aspirin.

6.45   Paracetamol toxicity is due to the formation of a reactive metabolite.

6.46   Indomethacin is a less effective anti-inflammatory drug than dextropropoxyphene.

6.47   Plasma levels of indomethacin may be reduced if probenecid is also taken.

6.48   Naproxen is free from gastrointestinal side effects.

6.49   Gold compounds are excreted within 24 hours of administration.

6.50   Therapy for patients with rheumatoid arthritis should be limited to a single medication.

6.51   Corticosteroids are drugs of choice as an initial drug treatment for arthritis.

6.52   Wound healing may be delayed by chronic use of corticosteroids.

6.53   Acute adrenal insufficiency may result from rapid withdrawal of chronic corticosteroid therapy.

6.54   Synthetic anti-inflammatory corticosteroids such as triamcinolone do not suppress the hypothalamic-pituitary-adrenal axis.

6.55   Probenecid, in small doses, may depress the excretion of uric acid.

6.56   For induction of labour at full term, ergotamine is preferable to prostaglandin $F_{2\alpha}$.

6.57   In the second trimester of pregnancy, uterine contraction is produced more effectively by prostaglandins than by ergotamine or oxytocin.

6.58   Intrauterine administration of prostaglandins is used to induce abortion.

6.59V   Luteolysis is the most useful veterinary property of prostaglandin $F_{2\alpha}$ and some of its synthetic analogues.

6.60   5-Hydroxytryptamine is formed by the hydroxylation and decarboxylation of tryptophan.

6.61   The major sites for 5-hydroxytryptamine storage in man are platelets and mast cells.

6.62   5-Hydroxytryptamine is broken down by enzymes in the liver.

6.63   5-Hydroxytryptamine is inactivated during passage through the pulmonary circulation.

6.64   Synthesis of 5-hydroxytryptamine is inhibited by methysergide.

6.65   There is now good evidence that all of the effects of 5-hydroxytryptamine in the periphery are mediated by either $5\text{-}HT_1$ or $5\text{-}HT_2$ receptors.

6.66   The presynaptic sympathetic inhibitory actions of 5-hydroxytryptamine are mediated by $5\text{-}HT_2$ receptors.

6.67   N-acetyl transferase is the enzyme involved in the conversion of angiotensin I to angiotensin II.

6.68   A brain renin-angiotensin system may play a role in the control of blood pressure.

6.69   Renin release from the kidney is stimulated by events which lower the blood pressure in the afferent arteriole.

6.70   Renin converts angiotensinogen to angiotensin I.

6.71   Circulating angiotensin II levels can be increased by salt depletion.

6.72   Captopril inhibits the conversion of angiotensin I to angiotensin II.

6.73   Saralasin is an angiotensin antagonist with some intrinsic activity.

6.74   Angiotensin increases blood pressure by acting on α-adrenoceptors.

6.75   Angiotensin II stimulates the release of aldosterone.

CORRECT OPTION

6.76 - 6.78

6.76   angiotensin

6.77   5-hydroxytryptamine

6.78   bradykinin

For each of the autacoids listed above, the major route of metabolism involves:

A.   an esterase
B.   a peptidase
C.   a monoamine oxidase
D.   a diamine oxidase
E.   a methyl transferase.

6.79   Histamine H_1-receptor antagonists:
A.   are the drugs of first choice in the treatment of anaphylactic reactions
B.   prevent the release of acid from the stomach
C.   reduce some inflammatory responses
D.   are free of side effects in therapeutic doses

6.80   Which of the following is least likely to result from administration of a histamine H_1-receptor antagonist?
A.   drowsiness
B.   relief of motion sickness
C.   inhibition of gastric acid secretion
D.   dryness of the mouth
E.   local anaesthesia.

6.81   Which of the following is not a histamine H_1-receptor antagonist?
A.   diphenhydramine
B.   dexchlorpheniramine
C.   phenylephrine
D.   promethazine
E.   cyclizine.

6.82   Histamine H_2-receptor antagonists are effective in the treatment of:
A.   angina
B.   peptic ulcer
C.   asthma
D.   dermatitis
E.   migraine.

6.83   Which of the following substances is not a pro-inflammatory mediator?
A.   adrenaline
B.   platelet activating factor
C.   leukotrienes
D.   bradykinin
E.   histamine.

6.84   Plasma kinins are formed following proteolysis of kininogens by:
    A.   kallidin
    B.   prekallikrein
    C.   kallikrein
    D.   kininases
    E.   aminopeptidase.

6.85   Bradykinin:
    A.   increases capillary permeability only in rodents
    B.   relaxes bronchial smooth muscle
    C.   relaxes vascular smooth muscle
    D.   relaxes uterine smooth muscle
    E.   produces pyrexia.

6.86   Arachidonic acid is:
    A.   only found in lung and renal tissue
    B.   the substrate for the synthesis of prostaglandin E_2
    C.   liberated from phospholipids before conversion to bradykinin
    D.   a small peptide comprising 20 amino acids
    E.   the stable biologically inactive metabolite of thromboxane A_2.

6.87   The metabolism of arachidonic acid by the lipoxygenase pathway:
    A.   is inhibited by indomethacin
    B.   leads to the biosynthesis of thromboxane A_2
    C.   is inhibited by histamine H_1-receptor antagonists
    D.   leads to the biosynthesis of leukotrienes
    E.   is responsible for intrinsic suppression of platelet aggregation.

6.88   Thromboxane A_2:
    A.   is released from endothelial cells
    B.   is derived from prostaglandin E_2
    C.   inhibits platelet aggregation
    D.   is degraded by enzymic action to thromboxane B_2
    E.   formation is inhibited by indomethacin.

6.89   Prostaglandins E_2 and I_2 :
    A.   are both circulating hormones
    B.   are excreted unchanged in the urine
    C.   potentiate the effects of histamine on vascular permeability
    D.   are systemic vasoconstrictors
    E.   are chemotactic for erythrocytes.

6.90   Leukotriene B_4:
    A.   is a biologically active peptide.
    B.   increases vascular permeability by a direct mechanism.
    C.   formation is inhibited by aspirin.
    D.   formation is inhibited by benoxaprofen.
    E.   suppresses the cellular response of inflammation.

6.91   Which of the following is chemotactic for polymorphonuclear leukocytes?
    A.   adrenaline
    B.   leukotriene B_4
    C.   GABA
    D.   5-hydroxytryptamine
    E.   leukotriene C_4.

6.92   Leukotriene D_4:
    A.   aggregates platelets
    B.   contracts airway smooth muscle
    C.   competitively antagonises the actions of isoprenaline at adrenergic receptors
    D.   inhibits prostaglandin synthesis
    E.   is chemotactic for polymorphonuclear leukocytes.

6.93   Which of the following drugs does not reduce prostaglandin formation by inhibiting cyclo-oxygenase or phospholipase A_2?
    A.   methysergide
    B.   aspirin
    C.   indomethacin
    D.   hydrocortisone
    E.   mepacrine.

6.94   Low-dose aspirin is used to treat atherosclerotic vascular disease because:
    A.   it facilitates the renal excretion of lipid peroxides
    B.   it is a vasodilator in the coronary circulation
    C.   it enhances prostacyclin release from the lungs
    D.   it has greater inhibitory effect on platelet cyclo-oxygenase than on endothelial cyclo-oxygenase
    E.   its lipolytic action decreases elevated plasma cholesterol.

6.95   Indomethacin inhibits the formation of:
    A.   histamine
    B.   leukotriene C
    C.   arachidonic acid
    D.   5-hydroxytryptamine
    E.   prostacyclin.

6.96   The anti-inflammatory action of nonsteroidal anti-inflammatory drugs may be attributed to:
    A.   antagonism of the effects of histamine via H_1-receptors
    B.   reduced synthesis of lipocortin
    C.   decreased tissue levels of arachidonic acid
    D.   inhibition of arachidonic acid metabolism via the cyclo-oxygenase pathway.
    E.   inhibition of the liberation of chemotactic factors.

6.97   In rheumatoid arthritis, the daily dose of aspirin for adults is approximately:
    A.   60 g
    B.   6 g
    C.   0.6 g
    D.   60 mg
    E.   6 mg.

6.98   The principal metabolite of a 300 mg dose of aspirin in man is:
    A.   salicylic acid
    B.   gentisic acid
    C.   salicyluric acid
    D.   acetylsalicylic acid.

6.99   Which of the following has the greatest protein binding?
        A.   aspirin
        B.   indomethacin
        C.   ibuprofen
        D.   chloroquine
        E.   prednisone.

6.100   In equipotent analgesic doses, which of the following drugs is the least
        effective anti-inflammatory agent?
        A.   aspirin
        B.   paracetamol
        C.   naproxen
        D.   indomethacin
        E.   salicylic acid.

6.101   Which of the following drugs is not used in the treatment of rheumatoid
        arthritis?
        A.   gold
        B.   penicillin
        C.   chloroquine
        D.   naproxen
        E.   prednisone.

6.102   The anti-inflammatory agent with the least incidence of toxicity is:
        A.   sodium aurothiomalate
        B.   chloroquine
        C.   D-penicillamine
        D.   naproxen.

6.103   The most frequent side effects of the nonsteroidal anti-inflammatory drugs
        involve the:
        A.   gastrointestinal tract
        B.   haematopoietic system
        C.   central nervous system
        D.   ear
        E.   eye.

6.104   Agranulocytosis is a side effect of:
        A.   theophylline
        B.   penicillamine
        C.   diazepam
        D.   insulin
        E.   digoxin.

6.105   Part of the anti-inflammatory effects of corticosteroids is due to:
        A.   stimulation of renin release from the kidney
        B.   increased synthesis of insulin in the pancreas
        C.   inhibition of phospholipase A_2 activity
        D.   decreased production of bradykinin from plasma kininogen
        E.   increased release of adrenocorticotrophic hormone from the
              pituitary gland.

6.106   Lipocortin mediates some of the anti-inflammatory effects of corticosteroids by:
    A.   inhibiting phospholipase A_2
    B.   antagonising the action of prostaglandin I_2 at receptor sites
    C.   increasing the formation of leukotriene B_4
    D.   stimulating chemokinesis
    E.   none of the above.

6.107   Part of the anti-inflammatory effect of chloroquine is due to:
    A.   lysis of macrophages
    B.   inhibition of phospholipase A_2 activity
    C.   antagonism of histamine H_1 receptors
    D.   inactivation of bradykinin.

6.108   Allopurinol lowers plasma uric acid concentrations by:
    A.   preventing active tubular reabsorption of uric acid
    B.   reducing the rate of conversion of xanthine to uric acid
    C.   increasing the glomerular filtration rate
    D.   decreasing levels of phosphoribosyl pyrophosphate synthetase
    E.   none of the above mechanisms.

6.109   Which of the following does not have 5-hydroxytryptamine antagonist activity?
    A.   pizotifen
    B.   ergotamine
    C.   methysergide
    D.   cyproheptadine
    E.   diphenhydramine.

6.110   Angiotensin II is:
    A.   a non-specific smooth muscle relaxant
    B.   a selective β_2-adrenoceptor agonist
    C.   a directly acting pressor agent
    D.   a monoamine oxidase inhibitor
    E.   an indirectly acting pressor agent.

6.111   The octapeptide angiotensin II:
    A.   is stored in the juxtaglomerular apparatus of the kidney
    B.   is antagonised by captopril
    C.   is a potent vasodilator
    D.   stimulates aldosterone release from the adrenal glands
    E.   is formed directly by the action of renin on an α-2 macroglobulin.

INCORRECT OPTION

6.112   Antigen-induced histamine release from mast cells:
    A.   involves a reduction in intracellular cyclic AMP levels
    B.   is a non-cytotoxic process
    C.   is independent of cellular energy metabolism
    D.   is suppressed by β-adrenoceptor agonists.

6.113 Capillary permeability in man is increased by:
    A. histamine
    B. 5-hydroxytryptamine
    C. bradykinin
    D. substance P
    E. platelet activating factor.

6.114 Increased vascular permeability:
    A. is caused by thromboxane A_2
    B. leads to oedema
    C. is caused by histamine
    D. due to bradykinin is enhanced by prostaglandin E_2
    E. in the inflammatory response is partly inhibited by mepyramine.

6.115 Both bradykinin and histamine:
    A. increase vascular permeability
    B. produce pain when applied to a blister base
    C. are mediators of inflammation
    D. have their biosynthesis inhibited by diphenhydramine
    E. dilate peripheral blood vessels.

6.116 Cyproheptadine:
    A. is used in the prophylaxis of migraine
    B. is a potent 5-hydroxytryptamine antagonist
    C. is a potent histamine H_1-receptor antagonist
    D. has no cranial vasoconstrictor activity at normal therapeutic doses
    E. can produce fibrosis.

6.117 Histamine:
    A. is formed from an amino acid by histidine decarboxylase
    B. increases vascular permeability
    C. is metabolised by monoamine oxidase
    D. is released in anaphylaxis.

6.118 Activation of histamine H_1-receptors produces:
    A. bronchial smooth muscle contraction
    B. gastrointestinal smooth muscle contraction
    C. increased capillary permeability
    D. dilation of arterioles
    E. positive inotropic effects in cardiac muscle.

6.119 Histamine H_1-receptor antagonists are therapeutically effective:
    A. in hay fever
    B. in urticaria
    C. in peptic ulcers
    D. as sedatives
    E. in motion sickness.

6.120 Cimetidine:
    A. blocks the action of histamine on bronchial smooth muscle
    B. blocks histamine H_2-receptors
    C. inhibits gastric acid secretion.

6.121 Promethazine has:
    A.   antiemetic properties
    B.   antipruritic properties
    C.   local anaesthetic activity
    D.   an inhibitory effect on gastric acid secretion
    E.   a phenothiazine structure.

6.122 The plasma kinins bradykinin and kallidin:
    A.   contain an identical nonapeptide moiety
    B.   are formed by a reaction pathway involving Hageman factor (clotting Factor XII)
    C.   are products of the proteolysis of kallikrein
    D.   have no recognised therapeutic uses
    E.   cannot be blocked by any specific competitive receptor antagonists.

6.123 Bradykinin:
    A.   increases capillary permeability
    B.   contracts bronchial smooth muscle
    C.   contracts uterine smooth muscle
    D.   may be involved in a variety of physiological vasoconstrictor functions
    E.   is not used therapeutically.

6.124 Bradykinin:
    A.   is extensively metabolised during a single passage through the pulmonary circulation
    B.   is a potent vasodilator
    C.   is synthesised from arachidonic acid
    D.   increases microvascular permeability
    E.   stimulates afferent pain fibres.

6.125 Methysergide:
    A.   is used in the prophylaxis of migraine
    B.   is a potent 5-hydroxytryptamine antagonist
    C.   is a potent histamine H_1-receptor antagonist
    D.   has no cranial vasoconstrictor activity at normal therapeutic doses
    E.   can produce fibrosis.

6.126 The involvement of prostaglandins and/or thromboxanes is likely to be important in:
    A.   parturition
    B.   platelet aggregation
    C.   malignant transformation of tumours
    D.   regulation of renal blood flow
    E.   central nervous system control of temperature.

6.127 Suppression of the formation of prostaglandins can be produced by:
    A.   aspirin
    B.   mepyramine
    C.   hydrocortisone
    D.   diethylcarbamazine
    E.   indomethacin.

6.128 Prostacyclin:
   A.   is not inactivated by prostaglandin dehydrogenase during a
        single passage through the pulmonary circulation
   B.   inhibits platelet aggregation
   C.   increases the levels of cyclic AMP in platelets
   D.   is metabolised to 6-keto prostaglandin $F_{1\alpha}$
   E.   is an inactive urinary metabolite of prostaglandin $F_{2\alpha}$.

6.129 Prostacyclin:
   A.   causes vasodilation
   B.   increases intracellular levels of cyclic AMP
   C.   inhibits platelet aggregation
   D.   induces bronchoconstriction
   E.   formation from arachidonic acid is inhibited by aspirin.

6.130 Both prostaglandin E_2 and prostaglandin $F_{2\alpha}$:
   A.   contract longitudinal smooth muscle in the gastrointestinal
        tract
   B.   are inactivated during passage through the pulmonary
        circulation
   C.   contract bronchial smooth muscle
   D.   cause decreased transit time in the intestine
   E.   cause diarrhoea.

6.131 Metabolites of a low dose of aspirin in man include:
   A.   salicylic acid
   B.   methyl salicylate
   C.   salicyluric acid
   D.   salicylic acid glucuronides.

6.132 The anti-inflammatory action of nonsteroidal anti-inflammatory drugs is
       due to:
   A.   inhibition of prostaglandin synthesis
   B.   stabilisation of endothelial cell membranes
   C.   scavenging of oxygen free radicals
   D.   inhibition of cell migration.

6.133 Renin is:
   A.   an endopeptidase
   B.   a steroid
   C.   released in response to a fall in blood pressure
   D.   found in normal plasma
   E.   synthesised in the kidney.

MCQ

6.134 Intradermal injections of histamine cause:
   i.   itching
   ii.   wheal
   iii. flare
   iv.   facial flushing
   v.   hypotension.

6.135 Which of the following drugs exhibit selectivity at histamine H_2-receptors?
    i.   diphenhydramine
    ii.   cimetidine
    iii. mepyramine
    iv. ranitidine
    v.   dexchlorpheniramine.

6.136 5-Hyroxytryptamine:
    i.   is synthesised in platelets
    ii.   synthesis is inhibited at the decarboxylation step by para-chlorophenylalanine
    iii. is metabolised by a diamine oxidase to 5-hydroxytryptophol
    iv. is actively taken up by platelets
    v.   uptake is unaffected by tricyclic antidepressants.

6.137 $5-HT_3$ receptors in the periphery mediate:
    i.   platelet aggregation
    ii.   stimulation of pain afferent fibres
    iii. relaxation of smooth muscle
    iv. activation of parasympathetic postganglionic neurones in the gastrointestinal tract.
    v.   vasoconstriction.

6.138 The anti-inflammatory action of corticosteroids:
    i.   is due to inhibition of phospholipase A_2
    ii.   requires the presence of a cell membrane receptor for corticosteroids
    iii. is inhibited by puromycin
    iv. is greatest in those steroids with most potent mineralocorticoid activity
    v.   occurs with physiological concentrations of hydrocortisone.

6.139 In acute inflammation:
    i.   vasodilation is the reason for the loss of function of an affected limb or organ
    ii.   swelling is largely due to macrophage accumulation
    iii. aspirin in low doses inhibits the lipoxygenase pathway of arachidonate metabolism
    iv. leukotriene B_4 is an important chemoattractant agent for polymorphs
    v.   prostaglandins prevent the pain induced by bradykinin.

6.140 Adrenaline is used in the emergency treatment of anaphylaxis because it:
    i.   stimulates cardiac β_1-adrenoceptors
    ii.   blocks α receptors in the peripheral arterioles
    iii. stimulates pulmonary β_2-adrenoceptors
    iv. reduces oxygen delivery to skeletal muscle
    v.   blocks prostaglandin release in the kidney.

ASSERTION / REASON

6.141 Antihistamines are the most effective drugs for treating motion sickness **BECAUSE** antihistamines act directly on the chemoreceptor trigger zone.

6.142 Cimetidine is used in the treatment of allergic dermatitis **BECAUSE** cimetidine blocks histamine H_2-receptors.

6.143　Diphenhydramine is an effective antipruritic agent **BECAUSE** diphenhydramine has both histamine H_1 - and H_2-receptor blocking properties.

6.144　Adrenaline is used in the treatment of acute anaphylactic shock **BECAUSE** adrenaline physiologically antagonises histamine-induced circulatory collapse.

6.145　Paracetamol in conventional therapeutic doses should not be given to patients with liver disease **BECAUSE** paracetamol in large doses causes hepatic liver necrosis.

6.146　Nonsteroidal anti-inflammatory drugs may cause gastric erosions **BECAUSE** nonsteroidal anti-inflammatory drugs inhibit the synthesis of prostaglandins.

6.147　Aspirin and indomethacin are anti-inflammatory drugs **BECAUSE** aspirin and indomethacin inhibit the synthesis of leukotrienes.

6.148　Corticosteroids are potent anti-inflammatory drugs **BECAUSE** corticosteroids inhibit the lipoxygenase pathway for the metabolism of arachidonic acid.

ANSWERS

6.1	F	6.26	F	6.51	F	6.76	B	6.101	B	6.126	C
6.2	T	6.27	T	6.52	T	6.77	C	6.102	D	6.127	B
6.3	T	6.28	F	6.53	T	6.78	B	6.103	A	6.128	E
6.4	F	6.29	T	6.54	F	6.79	C	6.104	B	6.129	D
6.5	F	6.30	T	6.55	T	6.80	C	6.105	C	6.130	C
6.6	T	6.31	T	6.56	F	6.81	C	6.106	A	6.131	B
6.7	T	6.32	F	6.57	T	6.82	B	6.107	B	6.132	B
6.8	T	6.33	T	6.58	T	6.83	A	6.108	B	6.133	B
6.9	T	6.34	T	6.59	T	6.84	C	6.109	E	6.134	A
6.10	T	6.35	T	6.60	T	6.85	C	6.110	C	6.135	C
6.11	F	6.36	F	6.61	F	6.86	B	6.111	D	6.136	D
6.12	F	6.37	F	6.62	T	6.87	D	6.112	C	6.137	C
6.13	T	6.38	T	6.63	T	6.88	E	6.113	B	6.138	B
6.14	T	6.39	F	6.64	F	6.89	C	6.114	A	6.139	D
6.15	T	6.40	T	6.65	F	6.90	D	6.115	D	6.140	B
6.16	F	6.41	F	6.66	F	6.91	B	6.116	E	6.141	C
6.17	F	6.42	F	6.67	F	6.92	B	6.117	C	6.142	D
6.18	T	6.43	F	6.68	T	6.93	A	6.118	E	6.143	C
6.19	T	6.44	F	6.69	T	6.94	D	6.119	C	6.144	A
6.20	T	6.45	T	6.70	T	6.95	E	6.120	A	6.145	D
6.21	F	6.46	F	6.71	T	6.96	D	6.121	D	6.146	A
6.22	F	6.47	F	6.72	T	6.97	B	6.122	C	6.147	C
6.23	F	6.48	F	6.73	T	6.98	C	6.123	D	6.148	C
6.24	T	6.49	F	6.74	F	6.99	C	6.124	C		
6.25	T	6.50	F	6.75	T	6.100	B	6.125	C		

7 Respiratory System

7.1 Histamine H_1-receptor antagonists can block histamine-induced bronchoconstriction.

7.2 Inositol triphosphate may be a second messenger for cholinergic agonists in airway smooth muscle.

7.3 Expectorant mucolytics increase the volume and decrease the viscosity of secretions in the respiratory tract.

7.4 Selective β_1-adrenoceptor agonists are beneficial in the treatment of bronchospasm.

7.5 β–Adrenoceptor antagonists may precipitate asthmatic attacks in susceptible individuals.

7.6 Disodium cromoglycate relaxes bronchial smooth muscle.

CORRECT OPTION

7.7 Which of the following drugs is not antitussive?
   A. noscapine
   B. nalorphine
   C. dextromethorphan
   D. codeine.

7.8 Which of the following compounds does not cause a rise in intracellular cyclic AMP levels in respiratory smooth muscle cells?
   A. orciprenaline
   B. terbutaline
   C. salbutamol
   D. propranolol

7.9 Which of the following drugs does not have agonist activity at β-adrenoceptors in respiratory smooth muscle?
   A. adrenaline
   B. isoprenaline
   C. terbutaline
   D. theophylline
   E. salbutamol.

7.10   Which of the following does not induce bronchospasm in asthmatics?
       A.   propranolol
       B.   atropine
       C.   sulphur dioxide
       D.   exercise
       E.   histamine.

7.11   Which of the following drug treatments is most useful in an acute attack of asthma?
       A.   beclomethasone aerosol
       B.   nebulised salbutamol
       C.   methacholine
       D.   chlorpheniramine
       E.   disodium cromoglycate.

7.12   Which of the following have been shown to inhibit both mediator release from lung tissue and relax respiratory smooth muscle tissue?
       A.   β-adrenoceptor agonists
       B.   disodium cromoglycate
       C.   histamine H_1-receptor antagonists
       D.   histamine H_2-receptor antagonists
       E.   corticosteroids.

7.13   Disodium cromoglycate:
       A.   is a bronchodilator
       B.   is useful in the treatment of an acute asthmatic attack
       C.   antagonises the effects of β-adrenoceptor antagonists
       D.   should be administered prophylactically.

7.14   Which of the following drug combinations should not be used for the treatment of asthma?
       A.   salbutamol and theophylline
       B.   disodium cromoglycate and salbutamol
       C.   beclomethasone dipropionate and terbutaline
       D.   salbutamol and ipratropium bromide
       E.   fenoterol and salbutamol.

7.15   Aerosol beclomethasone is an effective agent for the treatment of asthma because it:
       A.   suppresses the hypothalamic-pituitary-adrenal axis
       B.   releases catecholamines from the adrenal medulla
       C.   is a bronchodilator with a long duration of action
       D.   stimulates ciliary activity in respiratory epithelial cells
       E.   is a potent anti-inflammatory steroid.

7.16   Which of the following drugs will not inhibit the bronchoconstrictor response when given immediately before exercise in asthmatic subjects?
       A.   fenoterol
       B.   beclomethasone dipropionate
       C.   salbutamol
       D.   disodium cromoglycate.

7.17   Aspirin may precipitate asthma in sensitive subjects. The most likely explanation is that aspirin:
     A.   decreases the threshold of bronchial reactivity to prostaglandin $F_{2\alpha}$.
     B.   has β-adrenoceptor blocking activity
     C.   releases histamine from mast cells
     D.   increases the formation of leukotriene D in lung tissue
     E.   increases renal clearance of endogenous adrenaline.

7.18   Which of the following, administered *via* the airways, provides relief in acute attacks of asthma?
     A.   salbutamol
     B.   disodium cromoglycate
     C.   both drugs
     D.   neither drug.

7.19   Ipratropium bromide is useful in the treatment of asthma because it:
     A.   inhibits phosphodiesterase
     B.   stimulates β_2-adrenoceptors
     C.   inhibits the release of mast cell mediators
     D.   stimulates cholinergic receptors
     E.   none of the above.

INCORRECT OPTION

7.20   Drugs which are useful in the treatment of asthma include:
     A.   xanthine derivatives
     B.   calcium channel antagonists
     C. β_2-adrenoceptor agonists
     D.   disodium cromoglycate
     E.   aerosol corticosteroids.

7.21   In the treatment of asthma, β_2-adrenoceptor agonists:
     A.   relax bronchial smooth muscle
     B.   should not be administered to a patient taking corticosteroids
     C.   inhibit mediator release from mast cells
     D.   may be given orally, by aerosol or intravenously
     E.   exhibit some β_1-adrenoceptor agonist activity

MCQ

7.22   Disodium cromoglycate:
     i.   predisposes to oral candidiasis
     ii.   inhibits the metabolism of arachidonic acid *via* the lipoxygenase pathway
     iii.   causes bronchodilation
     iv.   blocks the bronchoconstrictor response to inhaled allergens
     v.   should not be prescribed for long term use.

7.23 Clinically effective doses of aerosol beclomethasone:
    i.   may predispose to oral candidiasis
    ii.   inhibit the hypothalamic-pituitary-adrenal axis
    iii. should be used by patients with suboptimal responses to bronchodilator therapy
    iv. inhibit immediate reactions to inhaled allergens
    v.   cause acute bronchodilation.

7.24 β-Adrenoceptor agonists:
    i.   inhibit antigen-antibody mediator release from lung tissue
    ii.   relax bronchial smooth muscle
    iii. competitively antagonise adenosine receptors
    iv. cause skeletal muscle tremor
    v.   stimulate the respiratory centre in the brain stem.

ASSERTION/REASON

7.25 Anticholinergic drugs are bronchodilators **BECAUSE** stimulation of the vagus nerve causes relaxation of airway smooth muscle.

7.26 β-Adrenoceptor agonists and anticholinergic drugs may be used in combination for the treatment of asthma **BECAUSE** both β–adrenoceptor agonists and anticholinergic drugs competitively antagonise histamine H_1 receptors.

ANSWERS

7.1	T	7.6	F	7.11	B	7.16	B	7.21	B	7.26	C
7.2	T	7.7	B	7.12	A	7.17	D	7.22	D		
7.3	T	7.8	D	7.13	D	7.18	A	7.23	B		
7.4	F	7.9	D	7.14	E	7.19	E	7.24	C		
7.5	T	7.10	B	7.15	E	7.20	B	7.25	C		

8 Cardiovascular System

TRUE / FALSE

8.1   The digitalis-induced diuresis observed in patients with congestive cardiac failure is due to a direct action of digitalis on the renal tubule.

8.2   Digoxin dosage should be reduced in patients with impaired renal function.

8.3   Digoxin is concentrated in cardiac muscle to levels considerably higher than those measured in plasma.

8.4   Severe congestive cardiac failure which does not respond to digoxin treatment may be reversed by combined vasodilator and dobutamine therapy.

8.5   Digitalis glycosides may control ventricular irregularities in patients with atrial flutter.

8.6   Amrinone is an inotropic agent with pronounced chronotropic activity.

8.7   Angiotensin converting enzyme inhibitors are useful in the treatment of congestive cardiac failure.

8.8   β-Adrenoceptor antagonists are useful in the treatment of arrhythmias due to digitalis overdose.

8.9   Antiarrhythmic agents cannot be used in combination to suppress arrhythmias.

8.10   All arrhythmias occurring shortly after a myocardial infarct are sensitive to lignocaine.

8.11   A solution of lignocaine containing adrenaline (10 g/ml) administered i.v. at 20 minute intervals is useful in controlling supraventricular tachycardia.

8.12   Lignocaine improves conduction in areas of unidirectional block.

8.13   Lignocaine metabolism is dependent on hepatic blood flow.

8.14   Mexiletine is an orally active antiarrhythmic agent.

8.15   Mexiletine, disopyramide and diltiazem are structurally related.

8.16   Lignocaine, mexiletine and tocainide are structurally related.

8.17   Verapamil and nifedipine have identical actions on calcium channels.

8.18   At therapeutic concentrations, verapamil exerts a greater antiarrhythmic effect than myocardial depressant effect.

8.19   The calcium channel blocking drugs (calcium antagonists) are effective in the management of atrial arrhythmias.

8.20   Drugs used in the treatment of angina are more rapidly effective if they are rubbed onto the skin than if they are taken sublingually.

8.21   Glyceryl trinitrate is rapidly absorbed from mucosal surfaces.

8.22   Glyceryl trinitrate tablets are taken sublingually to avoid irritant effects in the stomach.

8.23   The fall in blood pressure which occurs after taking glyceryl trinitrate reduces the work load and oxygen requirements of the heart.

8.24   The beneficial effect of glyceryl trinitrate in angina pectoris is due, at least in part, to a reduction of myocardial oxygen requirements.

8.25   The efficacy of glyceryl trinitrate in angina pectoris is due to its ability to dilate small coronary vessels.

8.26   Glyceryl trinitrate and propranolol are both useful for the treatment of angina.

8.27   β-Adrenoceptor blocking drugs are preferable to glyceryl trinitrate for the relief of an acute anginal attack.

8.28   Propranolol is of little use in the treatment of angina pectoris.

8.29   The cardiodepressant effect of propranolol can be reversed by verapamil.

Calcium antagonists used for the treatment of angina:

8.30   are specific antagonists of purinergic transmission.

8.31   inhibit smooth muscle contractions at lower concentrations than those which inhibit myocardial contractions.

8.32   are ineffective if the angina is due to coronary artery spasm.

8.33   The principal aim of the drug treatment of hypertension is to reduce complications of the disease.

8.34   Antihypertensive drugs reverse the underlying cause in essential hypertension.

8.35   Diuretics lower blood pressure by their actions in the central nervous system.

8.36   It is easier to maintain sodium depletion in the hypertensive patient with thiazide diuretics than by limitation of dietary salt.

8.37   Thiazide diuretics initially reduce blood pressure by reducing fluid volume.

8.38   Vasodilators alter blood flow in small vessels by reducing central sympathetic outflow.

8.39   Hydrallazine exerts its antihypertensive actions by blocking α-adrenoceptors.

8.40   The response to hydrallazine includes a reflex tachycardia.

8.41   Hydrallazine causes hypotension by a direct effect on vascular smooth muscle.

8.42   Prazosin and hydrallazine act by the same mechanism to lower blood pressure.

8.43   α-Methyldopa acts to lower blood pressure by blockade of postjunctional α-adrenoceptors.

8.44   The use of propranolol in hypertension is contraindicated in patients suffering from angina.

8.45   β-Adrenoceptor blocking drugs are especially useful in the treatment of patients with hypertension and cardiac failure.

8.46   The antihypertensive effect of clonidine is mediated *via* blockade of α_1-adrenoceptors.

8.47   Prazosin causes postural hypotension.

8.48   The hypotensive action of guanethidine is mediated by an inhibition of noradrenaline release.

8.49   The antihypertensive activity of guanethidine may be antagonised by tricyclic antidepressants.

8.50   Angiotensin converting enzyme inhibitors are useful in the treatment of high blood pressure.

8.51   Cough is a common side effect of angiotensin converting enzyme inhibitors.

8.52   Calcium channel blocking drugs decrease exercise capacity.

8.53   The effects of endothelium derived relaxant factor are mediated by intracellular increases in cyclic GMP.

8.54   All diuretics act by increasing sodium reabsorption in the renal tubules.

8.55   Most diuretics cause an increase in urine flow by increasing the glomerular filtration rate.

8.56   The hypotensive effects of the thiazide diuretics are related to potassium loss.

8.57   The diuretic effect of chlorothiazide is independent of acid-base balance.

8.58   Frusemide causes a diuresis characterised by a high level of sodium excretion accompanied by a low level of potassium and bicarbonate excretion.

8.59   An osmotic diuretic is a non-electrolyte which is filtered at the glomerulus and undergoes minimal reabsorption.

8.60   Vasopressin increases the permeability of the tubular cells to Na^+ at the distal and collecting tubules.

8.61   Vasopressin causes diuresis by increasing the absorption of Cl^-.

8.62   Warfarin inhibits vitamin K-dependent synthesis of prothrombin in the liver.

8.63   Warfarin is only effective if administered by intravenous injection.

8.64   Protamine sulphate is indicated in the treatment of warfarin overdose.

8.65   Vitamin K_1 is used in the treatment of haemorrhage due to warfarin overdose.

8.66   Plasmin is a proteolytic enzyme which accelerates the formation of angiotensin.

8.67   Sodium citrate is the anticoagulant used most commonly by blood banks when storing blood for transfusion.

8.68   Prevention of coagulation by citrate ions does not preclude the use of blood for transfusions.

8.69   Antagonism of heparin overdose cannot be accomplished in less than 12 hours.

8.70   Long-term salicylate therapy enhances blood coagulation.

8.71   Patients on oral anticoagulant therapy should take aspirin in preference to paracetamol as an antipyretic analgesic.

8.72   Oral administration of iron preparations is associated with a greater incidence of side effects than parenteral administration.

8.73   Macrocytic anaemias, other then pernicious anaemia, generally respond to therapy with folic acid.

8.74   For treating anaemias, folic acid should not be given alone unless a vitamin B_{12} deficiency has been excluded.

8.75 V Orally administered organic salts of iron are the drugs of choice in the treatment of piglet anaemia.

8.76   Nicotinamide is a useful hypolipidaemic agent.

8.77   The hypocholesterolaemic activity of clofibrate is largely due to effects on hepatic intermediary metabolism.

8.78   Sitosterols reduce the absorption of both exogenous and endogenous cholesterol.

8.79   All the known metabolic effects of cholestyramine are directly or indirectly related to the sequestration of bile acids.

CORRECT OPTION

8.80-8.82

8.80   propranolol

8.81   glyceryl trinitrate

8.82   metoprolol

For each of the drugs above, indicate whether it:

A.   is used in the acute management of an anginal attack
B.   is a selective β_1-adrenoceptor blocker, useful in the treatment of hypertension
C.   is a centrally-acting α-adrenoceptor stimulant, useful in the treatment of hypertension
D.   is a non-selective β-adrenoceptor blocker, useful in the treatment of angina
E.   lowers blood pressure by adrenergic neurone blockade.

8.83   The positive inotropic action of digoxin
A.   is blocked by propranolol
B.   depends upon elevation of cardiac cyclic-AMP levels
C.   requires its active transport into the cardiac cell
D.   arises from an increased intracellular concentration of calcium ions
E.   is abolished by prior reserpinisation.

8.84   A major biochemical effect of cardiac glycosides is:
A.   enhancement of cardiac ribosome function in protein synthesis
B.   enhancement of muscarinic receptor function in the heart
C.   inhibition of acetylcholinesterase
D.   inhibition of monoamine oxidase
E.   inhibition of Na^+,K^+-stimulated ATPase.

8.85   The antiarrhythmic actions of:
A.   quinidine are partly due to its ability to prolong the refractory period of heart muscle
B.   quinidine are accompanied by a cardiac stimulant action
C.   procainamide are of shorter duration than those of procaine
D.   propranolol are due to its local anaesthetic activity
E.   verapamil are associated with β-adrenoceptor blockade.

8.86 Glyceryl trinitrate:
  A. has a direct stimulant effect on the myocardium
  B. is useful in the treatment of myasthenia gravis
  C. causes generalised smooth muscle relaxation
  D. often produces a bradycardia
  E. is a calcium channel antagonist.

8.87 β-Adrenoceptor antagonists are frequently used with thiazide diuretics because:
  A. the diuretics elevate plasma lipids
  B. the diuretics counter the fall in plasma potassium produced by the β-adrenoceptor antagonists
  C. their antihypertensive actions are synergistic
  D. both drugs slow the heart
  E. thiazides alter the excretion of the β-adrenoceptor antagonists.

8.88 α-Methyldopa exerts its antihypertensive action through:
  A. blockade of β-adrenoceptors
  B. stimulation of prejunctional β-adrenoceptors
  C. blockade of prejunctional α-adrenoceptors
  D. stimulation of central α-adrenoceptors
  E. combined α- and β-adrenoceptor blockade.

8.89 Which of the following does not cause contraction of vascular smooth muscle?
  A. noradrenaline
  B. angiotensin
  C. adrenaline
  D. glyceryl trinitrate
  E. vasopressin.

8.90 Adenosine causes vasoconstriction of the blood vessels in:
  A. brain
  B. adipose tissue
  C. kidney
  D. heart
  E. skeletal muscle.

8.91 Which of the following does not stimulate release of endothelium derived relaxant factor?
  A. acetylcholine
  B. glyceryl trinitrate
  C. histamine
  D. hydrallazine
  E. vasoactive intestinal peptide.

8.92 Mannitol may be classified as:
  A. an acidifying diuretic
  B. a carbonic anhydrase inhibitor
  C. an osmotic diuretic
  D. a loop diuretic
  E. a distal tubule diuretic.

8.93   Tolerance to the action of carbonic anhydrase inhibitors may arise because
        they cause loss of:
        A.   bicarbonate in the urine and a metabolic alkalosis
        B.   bicarbonate in the urine and a metabolic acidosis
        C.   chloride in the urine and a metabolic alkalosis
        D.   chloride in the urine and a metabolic acidosis.

8.94   Acetazolamide is a diuretic because:
        A.   it inhibits carbonic anhydrase in the epithelial cells of the
              proximal tubule
        B.   it inhibits sodium transport in the distal tubule
        C.   it increases the active transport of water in the distal tubule
        D.   it stimulates Na^+,K^+-ATPase
        E.   none of the above.

8.95   The primary mechanism of the diuretic action of spironolactone depends
        on its ability to:
        A.   antagonise the action of vasopressin (ADH)
        B.   suppress the release of vasopressin from the posterior pituitary
        C.   suppress the release of aldosterone from the adrenal cortex
        D.   competitively antagonise the action of aldosterone
        E   inhibit the enzyme carbonic anhydrase.

8.96   Which of the following drugs is likely to cause the greatest increase in
        urinary pH?
        A.   urea
        B.   frusemide
        C.   ethanol
        D.   acetazolamide
        E.   fludrocortisone.

8.97   Which of the following diuretics is contraindicated in the presence of
        hyperkalaemia?
        A.   acetazolamide
        B.   chlorothiazide
        C.   ethacrynic acid
        D.   frusemide
        E.   spironolactone.

8.98   Which of the following acts as a diuretic by depressing the release of
        antidiuretic hormone?
        A.   frusemide
        B.   ethanol
        C.   urea
        D.   spironolactone
        E.   acetazolamide.

8.99   Frusemide:
        A.   causes Na^+, K^+, Cl^- and water loss and may produce alkalosis
        B.   causes Na^+, K^+, Cl^- and water loss without affecting acid-base
              balance
        C.   causes Na^+, K^+, HCO_3^- and water loss and may produce acidosis
        D.   causes Na^+, Cl^- and water loss, without affecting K^+ excretion
              and antagonises aldosterone
        E.   none of the above.

Cardiovascular System

8.100-8.103

8.100   inhibits Cl⁻ absorption in the loop of Henle

8.101   inhibits HCO₃⁻ reabsorption, causes a metabolic acidosis

8.102   inhibits Na⁺ reabsorption distally, conserves K⁺, but does not antagonise aldosterone

8.103   inhibits Na⁺ reabsorption distally, conserves K⁺ and antagonises aldosterone

For each of the descriptions above, indicate whether it applies to:

A.   acetazolamide
B.   triamterene
C.   chlorothiazide
D.   ethacrynic acid
E.   spironolactone.

8.104-8.105

8.104   most likely to cause hypokalaemia

8.105   induces a diuresis by depressing the release of vasopressin

For each of the descriptions above, indicate whether it applies to:

A.   frusemide
B.   acetazolamide
C.   spironolactone
D.   urea
E.   ethanol.

8.106   The most important action of heparin when used as an anticoagulant is its ability to:
A.   chelate calcium ions
B.   inhibit production of Factors VII, IX and X
C.   induce platelet aggregation
D.   inhibit fibrinogen polymerisation.

8.107   Heparin:
A.   is effective when administered by mouth
B.   is quickly inactivated by enzymes
C.   is safe in haemophiliacs
D.   decreases the blood viscosity
E.   is rapidly antagonised by protein sulphates.

8.108   Heparin:
A.   prevents the synthesis of prothrombin
B.   delays the conversion of prothrombin to thrombin
C.   acts by chelating calcium
D.   delays the conversion of fibrin to fibrinogen
E.   is administered by intramuscular injection.

8.109　Which of the following is capable of combining with heparin so as to render it biologically inactive?
- A. protamine
- B. inositol
- C. histidine
- D. cephalin
- E. alanine.

8.110　Warfarin is an anticoagulant which acts by:
- A. precipitating calcium ions
- B. directly inhibiting prothrombin conversion to thrombin
- C. depolymerising fibrin
- D. disaggregating platelets
- E. inhibiting formation of vitamin K-dependent co-factors.

8.111　Which of the following improves megaloblastic anaemia but does not protect against the neurologic manifestations of pernicious anaemia?
- A. vitamin K
- B. folic acid
- C. vitamin B_{12}
- D. niacin
- E. thiamine.

8.112　Clofibrate:
- A. lowers plasma triglyceride levels to a greater extent than plasma cholesterol levels
- B. has been clearly shown to prevent death from coronary artery disease
- C. impairs the absorption of fat-soluble vitamins
- D. is a synonym for colestipol
- E. is poorly absorbed from the gastrointestinal tract.

INCORRECT OPTION

8.113　Calcium antagonists are useful in the treatment of:
- A. high blood pressure
- B. tremor
- C. tachyarrhythmias
- D. angina.

8.114　The positive inotropic action of digitalis:
- A. has been demonstrated in isolated strips of heart muscle
- B. is independent of the central nervous system
- C. is not due to prolongation of the contractile process
- D. occurs despite shortening of the systolic time
- E. can be inhibited by α-adrenoceptor antagonists.

8.115　Structural requirements for optimal activity in cardiac glycosides include:
- A. an unsaturated lactone ring
- B. a near-planar steroid nucleus
- C. sugar molecules
- D. hydroxyl groups on the steroid nucleus.

8.116   Cardiac arrhythmias may be suppressed by:
        A.   atropine
        B.   verapamil
        C.   amitriptyline
        D.   mexiletine
        E.   amiodarone.

8.117   Indications for cardiac glycoside therapy include:
        A.   atrial fibrillation
        B.   congestive cardiac failure
        C.   ventricular bradycardia
        D.   atrial flutter.

8.118   In effective antiarrhythmic doses, quinidine may:
        A.   cause tachycardia
        B.   cause tinnitus
        C.   have a positive inotropic action
        D.   increase the relative refractory period of the cardiac muscle
        E.   depress the automaticity of the cardiac muscle.

8.119   Vasodilators may prevent or reduce attacks of angina because they:
        A.   reverse coronary artery spasm
        B.   reduce venous return and end diastolic volume
        C.   cause coronary vasodilation
        D.   reduce the work performed by the heart
        E.   reduce heart rate.

8.120   Both propranolol and glyceryl trinitrate:
        A.   are effective antiarrhythmic agents
        B.   are subject to extensive first pass metabolism
        C.   are effective in the treatment of angina pectoris
        D.   have some hypotensive activity.

8.121   Clonidine treatment:
        A.   is effective because of stimulation of central α-adrenoceptors
        B.   may be associated with acute hypertension
        C.   is accompanied by a fall in sympathetic outflow
        D.   may cause nasal stuffiness
        E.   is the treatment of choice in alcoholic hypertensives.

8.122   β-Adrenoceptor blocking drugs are effective antihypertensive agents because they:
        A.   reduce cardiac output
        B.   block β-adrenergic effects in the muscle vasculature
        C.   reduce central sympathetic outflow
        D.   depress the activity of the renin-angiotensin-aldosterone system.

8.123   Vasoconstriction may be reduced by:
        A.   hydrallazine
        B.   papaverine
        C.   angiotensin II
        D.   prazosin
        E.   verapamil.

8.124   In diuretic therapy:
    A.   fruit such as oranges and pineapples can be used as a potassium supplement
    B.   it is not necessary to give potassium supplements to patients taking spironolactone
    C.   chlorothiazide may cause gout
    D.   hypokalaemia is a major problem in patients taking frusemide
    E.   acetazolamide causes an increase in the excretion of K^+ but not of Na^+.

8.125   The anticoagulant activity of heparin is associated with:
    A.   prolongation of activated partial thromboplastin time
    B.   suppression of the formation of clotting factors
    C.   a variable effect on platelet function
    D.   inhibition of thrombin formation.

8.126   Warfarin:
    A.   in the plasma is mostly protein bound
    B.   decreases the formation of prothrombin
    C.   may be potentiated by phenylbutazone
    D.   is active both *in vivo* and *in vitro*
    E.   has been used as a rodenticide.

8.127   Iron deficiency is commonly treated by:
    A.   ferrous sulphate
    B.   ferrous chloride
    C.   ferrous fumarate
    D.   ferrous gluconate
    E.   ferrous carbonate.

8.128   Concerning iron absorption and requirements:
    A.   Women's daily requirements are greater than men's.
    B.   There is an increased requirement during pregnancy.
    C.   Iron in the ferric state is more readily absorbed.
    D.   Iron is stored in a protein-bound form as ferritin.
    E.   An iron deficient person usually absorbs iron more efficiently than when iron stores are normal.

8.129   Iron absorption from the gastrointestinal tract is:
    A.   enhanced by hydrochloric acid in the gastric juice
    B.   greater when iron is in the ferrous form
    C.   greater when iron is in the form of a succinate rather then a phytate
    D.   maximal in the large intestine
    E.   predominantly by means of a regulated active uptake process.

MCQ

8.130   Which of the following are side effects of digoxin?
    i.   cardiac arrhythmias
    ii.   fluid retention
    iii.   nausea and vomiting
    iv.   haemolytic anaemia
    v.   thrombocytopaenia.

8.131   Which of the following drugs, when administered concurrently alter(s) digoxin plasma concentration?
     i.   amiodarone
     ii.   quinidine
     iii. verapamil
     iv. lignocaine
     v.   mexiletine.

8.132   β-Adrenoceptor antagonists are useful in the treatment of:
     i.   high blood pressure
     ii.   tremor
     iii. tachyarrhythmias
     iv. congestive heart failure
     v.   stroke.

8.133   i.   All cardiac glycosides contain a steroid ring.
     ii.   Many cardiac glycosides are synthetic substances.
     iii. All cardiac glycosides contain a lactone ring.
     iv. Digitoxin is not a cardiac glycoside.
     v.   Clinically useful cardiac glycosides can be extracted from oleander plants.

8.134   Which of the following is/are useful in the treatment of congestive heart failure?
     i.   digoxin
     ii.   vasodilators
     iii. α-adrenoceptor antagonists
     iv. diuretics
     v.   angiotensin converting enzyme inhibitors.

8.135   Procainamide and quinidine:
     i.   are structurally related
     ii.   have similar membrane actions, leading to decrease responsiveness and decreased automaticity
     iii. are both metabolised in the liver by the same pathway
     iv. both have short half-lives and therefore need to be given at frequent intervals
     v.   both alter the kinetics of digoxin, leading to increased plasma concentrations of that drug.

8.136   Which of the following enhance conduction through an area of unidirectional block?
     i.   propranolol
     ii.   lignocaine
     iii. quinidine
     iv. phenytoin
     v.   hypoxia.

8.137   Which of the following is useful in the treatment of angina pectoris?
     i.   verapamil
     ii.   glyceryl trinitrate
     iii. propranolol
     iv. digoxin
     v.   dobutamine.

8.138   β-Adrenoceptor blocking drugs are useful in angina pectoris because they:
    i.   reduce heart rate responses
    ii.   unmask α-adrenoceptor effects
    iii. reduce myocardial oxygen demands
    iv. limit respiratory performance
    v.   are potent local anaesthetics.

8.139   Vasodilators:
    i.   act on prejunctional α-adrenoceptors and reduce sympathetic tone
    ii.   act on arteries to reduce afterload
    iii. act through inhibition of phosphodiesterase
    iv. act on veins to reduce preload
    v.   may induce coronary vasospasm through purinergic mechanisms.

8.140   Prazosin:
    i.   has a greater hypotensive effect in salt-depleted patients
    ii.   inhibits noradrenaline release
    iii. may cause severe postural hypotension
    iv. selectively blocks α_2-adrenoceptors
    v.   is a potent phosphodiesterase inhibitor at therapeutic plasma concentrations.

8.141   Angiotensin converting enzyme inhibitors lower blood pressure:
    i.   to a greater extent in the presence of salt depletion
    ii.   to a limited extent in all subjects
    iii. through changes in levels of kinins and angiotensin II
    iv. only in conjunction with a centrally acting drug
    v.   in rats but not in man.

8.142   Angiotensin converting enzyme inhibitors can cause an exaggerated fall in blood pressure when the subject:
    i.   has been taking a low salt diet
    ii.   is taking other drugs which block sympathetic reflexes
    iii. is taking a diuretic
    iv. is aged 75 years or more
    v.   has a significant renal artery stenosis.

8.143   β-Adrenoceptor blocking drugs are effective antihypertensive drugs because they:
    i.   block cardiac β-adrenoceptors
    ii.   increase the force of contraction of the myocardium
    iii. reduce vascular responsiveness
    iv. block β-adrenoceptors in the muscle vascular bed
    v.   increase central sympathetic effects.

8.144   Calcium antagonists:
    i.   are specific antagonists of purinergic transmission
    ii.   inhibit smooth muscle contraction
    iii. inhibit skeletal muscle contraction
    iv. improve myocardial metabolism during myocardial ischaemia
    v.   prevent formation of renal calculi.

8.145   Calcium antagonists:
    i.   have widely different molecular structures
    ii.   slow A-V nodal conduction in the heart
    iii. lower blood pressure
    iv. may be effective in the treatment of supraventricular tachycardia
    v.   affect voltage-dependent channels in cell membranes.

8.146   The diuretic actions of chlorothiazide include:
    i.   increased excretion of Na^+
    ii.   increased excretion of K^+
    iii. increased excretion of Cl^-
    iv. antagonism of the effects of aldosterone
    v.   inhibition of ADH release.

8.147   Thiazide diuretics:
    i.   increase sodium and water excretion
    ii.   produce hypokalaemia
    iii. reduce blood volume and cardiac output
    iv. reduce plasma concentrations of uric acid
    v.   reduce plasma renin concentrations.

8.148   Which of the following are potassium sparing diuretics?
    i.   trimipramine
    ii.   spironolactone
    iii. ethacrynic acid
    iv. amiloride
    v.   frusemide.

8.149   All potassium sparing diuretics:
    i.   work by the same mechanism
    ii.   inhibit carbonic anhydrase
    iii. antagonise aldosterone
    iv. may cause hyperkalaemia
    v.   are very potent diuretics.

8.150   Which of the following statements concerning the oral anticoagulants, coumarin and phenindione, is/are true?
    i.   Their rate of onset of action depends on hepatic stores of vitamin K.
    ii.   They are extensively metabolised by hepatic microsomal enzymes.
    iii. Their action on vitamin K-dependent factors is exerted principally through Factor V.
    iv. They can be displaced from plasma protein binding sites by a number of drugs.
    v.   Adequate anticoagulant control can best be achieved by repeated measurements of plasma drug concentrations.

8.151   Heparin:
    i.   is inactivated by protamine sulphate
    ii.   activates lipoprotein lipase
    iii. requires a cofactor (antithrombin III) for its anticoagulant effect
    iv. is extracted from the venom of the Malayan pit-viper
    v.   is well absorbed after oral administration.

8.152 Which of the following are potentially hazardous in patients taking oral anticoagulants?
    i.   amoxycillin
    ii.   phenylbutazone
    iii. acetylsalicylic acid
    iv. oxazepam
    v.   paracetamol.

ASSERTION/REASON

8.153 Angiotensin converting enzyme inhibitors are useful in the treatment of congestive heart failure **BECAUSE** converting enzyme inhibitors reduce plasma renin activity.

8.154 Digoxin slows conduction through the atrio-ventricular node **BECAUSE** digoxin abolishes spontaneous diastolic depolarisation (Phase 4).

8.155 Verapamil is widely used for the treatment of atrial tachyarrhythmias **BECAUSE** verapamil blocks the inward flux of Ca^{2+} in vascular smooth muscle.

8.156 β-Adrenoceptor antagonists and calcium antagonists have no additive effects on myocardial performance **BECAUSE** their actions are mediated by separate and discrete pathways.

8.157 Procaine is widely used as an antiarrhythmic agent **BECAUSE** procaine has membrane-stabilising properties.

8.158 Tocainide is active after oral administration **BECAUSE** tocainide is not metabolised to any extent by the liver.

8.159 Lignocaine is given in the pre-hospital treatment of myocardial infarction **BECAUSE** lignocaine is a potent local anaesthetic.

8.160 Glyceryl trinitrate reduces the symptoms of angina pectoris **BECAUSE** glyceryl trinitrate reduces venous return and reverses coronary spasm if it is present.

8.161 Glyceryl trinitrate relieves coronary artery spasm **BECAUSE** glyceryl trinitrate blocks 5-HT receptors in the coronary vasculature.

8.162 Glyceryl trinitrate is used prophylactically in patients with angina **BECAUSE** glyceryl trinitrate is rapidly absorbed through the buccal mucosa.

8.163 Calcium channel blocking drugs are of limited use in angina pectoris **BECAUSE** when combined with β-adrenoceptor blocking drugs, calcium channel blocking drugs may cause marked cardiac depression.

8.164 The treatment of mild hypertension produces little or no reduction in heart disease **BECAUSE** the treatment of mild hypertension frequently alters lipid levels.

8.165 Hydrallazine and prazosin may have additive effects in the treatment of hypertension **BECAUSE** hydrallazine and prazosin act at separate sites on the vascular smooth muscle.

8.166 Abrupt clonidine withdrawal may cause marked hypertension **BECAUSE** abrupt clonidine withdrawal is associated with a sudden increase in the release of noradrenaline.

8.167 Dopamine increases renal blood flow **BECAUSE** dopamine stimulates the force of contraction of the heart.

8.168 Amiloride is often administered with thiazide diuretics **BECAUSE** amiloride promotes the excretion of potassium.

8.169 Amiloride is a potassium-sparing diuretic **BECAUSE** amiloride acts in the distal convoluted tubule to inhibit Na^+/K^+ exchange.

8.170 Salt and water loss enhance the effects of converting enzyme inhibitors **BECAUSE** salt and water loss increases the dependence of the blood pressure control systems on angiotensin.

8.171 Adenosine increases blood pressure **BECAUSE** adenosine dilates coronary arteries.

ANSWERS

8.1	F	8.32	F	8.63	F	8.94	A	8.125	B	8.156	D
8.2	T	8.33	T	8.64	F	8.95	D	8.126	D	8.157	D
8.3	T	8.34	F	8.65	T	8.96	D	8.127	B	8.158	C
8.4	T	8.35	F	8.66	F	8.97	E	8.128	C	8.159	B
8.5	T	8.36	T	8.67	T	8.98	B	8.129	D	8.160	A
8.6	F	8.37	T	8.68	T	8.99	A	8.130	B	8.161	C
8.7	T	8.38	F	8.69	F	8.100	D	8.131	C	8.162	B
8.8	T	8.39	F	8.70	F	8.101	A	8.132	A	8.163	D
8.9	F	8.40	T	8.71	F	8.102	B	8.133	B	8.164	A
8.10	F	8.41	T	8.72	T	8.103	E	8.134	E	8.165	A
8.11	F	8.42	F	8.73	T	8.104	A	8.135	C	8.166	A
8.12	T	8.43	F	8.74	T	8.105	E	8.136	C	8.167	B
8.13	T	8.44	F	8.75	F	8.106	D	8.137	A	8.168	C
8.14	T	8.45	F	8.76	F	8.107	B	8.138	B	8.169	A
8.15	F	8.46	F	8.77	T	8.108	B	8.139	C	8.170	A
8.16	T	8.47	T	8.78	T	8.109	A	8.140	B	8.171	D
8.17	F	8.48	T	8.79	T	8.110	E	8.141	A		
8.18	T	8.49	T	8.80	D	8.111	B	8.142	E		
8.19	T	8.50	T	8.81	A	8.112	A	8.143	B		
8.20	F	8.51	T	8.82	B	8.113	B	8.144	C		
8.21	T	8.52	F	8.83	D	8.114	E	8.145	E		
8.22	F	8.53	T	8.84	E	8.115	B	8.146	A		
8.23	T	8.54	F	8.85	A	8.116	C	8.147	A		
8.24	T	8.55	F	8.86	C	8.117	C	8.148	C		
8.25	F	8.56	F	8.87	C	8.118	C	8.149	C		
8.26	T	8.57	T	8.88	D	8.119	E	8.150	C		
8.27	F	8.58	F	8.89	D	8.120	B	8.151	A		
8.28	F	8.59	T	8.90	C	8.121	E	8.152	A		
8.29	F	8.60	F	8.91	B	8.122	B	8.153	C		
8.30	F	8.61	F	8.92	C	8.123	C	8.154	C		
8.31	T	8.62	T	8.93	B	8.124	E	8.155	B		

9 Gastrointestinal Tract

TRUE / FALSE

9.1   In an antacid mixture, the constipating effects of aluminium salts can be offset by the purgative action of magnesium salts.

9.2   Aluminium toxicity may be a side effect of antacid therapy.

9.3   Omeprazole blocks gastric acid secretion by a mechanism which does not involve histamine H_2 receptors.

9.4   Dioctyl sodium sulphosuccinate produces its laxative effects by stimulating colonic smooth muscle.

9.5   Bisacodyl is a bulk laxative.

9.6   Quaternary ammonium anticholinergics are the drugs of choice for the control of diarrhoea.

9.7   The antispasmodic activity of mebeverine results from antagonist activity at muscarinic receptors.

9.8V   Poloxalene can be given prophylactically to prevent bloat in cattle.

9.9V   Apomorphine acts as an emetic in the dog by stimulating the vomiting centre in the medulla.

9.10   The antiemetic effect of chlorcyclizine is partly due to its anticholinergic activity.

9.11   The antiemetic response to neuroleptics involves an action at the basal ganglia.

9.12V   Benzodiazepines are useful for prophylactic treatment for motion sickness in cats and dogs.

CORRECT OPTION

9.13   Which of the following is not used as an antacid?
  A.   aluminium hydroxide
  B.   calcium carbonate
  C.   magnesium trisilicate
  D.   sodium bicarbonate
  E.   sodium metabisulphite.

9.14   Which of the following is the most suitable laxative for an elderly person?
    A.   phenolphthalein
    B.   castor oil
    C.   magnesium sulphate
    D.   liquid paraffin
    E.   bran.

9.15   The laxative action of danthron is due to:
    A.   formation of irritant fatty acids
    B.   stimulation of local afferent nerve fibres
    C.   its hygroscopic properties
    D.   its hypertonicity
    E.   none of the above.

9.16   Which of the following drugs is not effective in the treatment of peptic ulcers?
    A.   carbenoxolone sodium
    B.   cimetidine
    C.   phenylbutazone
    D.   ranitidine
    E.   tripotassium dicitrato bismuthate.

9.17   Which of the following does not commonly cause constipation?
    A.   codeine
    B.   amoxycillin
    C.   atropine
    D.   verapamil.

9.18   Which of the following drugs does not commonly cause nausea and vomiting?
    A.   digoxin
    B.   cimetidine
    C.   fluorouracil
    D.   ipecacuanha
    E.   morphine.

9.19   Which of the following is not used as an antiemetic?
    A.   chlorpromazine
    B.   Δ-9-tetrahydrocannabinol
    C.   diphenhydramine
    D.   metoclopramide
    E.   oxazepam.

9.20-9.21

9.20   carbenoxolone

9.21   ipecacuanha

For each of the drugs above indicate whether it:

    A.   is principally a centrally acting emetic
    B.   is a reflex emetic with weak centrally mediated emetic properties
    C.   increases the rate of healing of peptic ulcers
    D.   is a synthetic anthraquinone derivative
    E.   is none of the above.

9.22V   Which of the following drugs is not used as an anticoccidial agent for poultry?
    A.   amprolium
    B.   clopidol
    C.   sodium arsenilate
    D.   sulphaquinoxaline
    E.   robenidine.

9.23V   Which of the following is the least safe drug to use for the treatment of frothy bloat in cattle?
    A.   liquid paraffin
    B.   oil of turpentine
    C.   alcohol ethoxylates
    D.   poloxalene
    E.   dioctyl sodium sulphosuccinate.

INCORRECT OPTION:

9.24V   Concerning emetic agents:
    A.   If a first dose of apomorphine is ineffective, then further doses are less likely to result in vomiting.
    B.   Apomorphine stimulates central dopamine receptors.
    C.   Metoclopramide produces emesis *via* an effect on the gastrointestinal tract.
    D.   Ipecacuanha acts principally by peripheral gastric irritation.
    E.   In cats, xylazine produces emesis followed by sedation.

9.25   In the gastrointestinal tract, morphine:
    A.   increases the rate of gastric emptying
    B.   increases the background tone of the small and large intestines
    C.   decreases propulsive peristalsis
    D.   increases absorption of water from the intestinal contents
    E.   increases the tone of the anal sphincter.

9.26   Diphenoxylate:
    A.   has less risk of dependence than morphine
    B.   is hydrolysed in the intestine to ricinoleic acid
    C.   increases muscular tone of the anal sphincter
    D.   decreases gastrointestinal motility
    E.   is structurally related to pethidine.

9.27   Metoclopramide:
    A.   increases gastric peristalsis
    B.   has a laxative action
    C.   antagonises the action of dopamine
    D.   raises the threshold of the chemoreceptor trigger zone
    E.   has an antiemetic action.

MCQ

9.28   Which of the following are used in the treatment of peptic ulcers?
     i.   antacids and cimetidine
     ii.   simple dietary measures and alteration in life style
     ii.   bismuth-containing mixtures
     iv. selective histamine H_1-receptor antagonists
     v.   pentagastrin and cimetidine.

9.29   Which of the following drugs delay gastric emptying?
     i.   metoclopramide
     ii.   probanthine
     iii. cimetidine
     iv. amitryptiline
     v.   digoxin.

9.30   Which of the following are useful in the treatment of diarrhoea?
     i.   codeine
     ii.   loperamide
     iii. diphenoxylate
     iv. phenolphthalein
     v.   dioctyl sodium sulphosuccinate.

9.31   Diphenoxylate is effective in the treatment of diarrhoea because:
     i.   it is an anticholinergic
     ii.   it is a synthetic congener of cocaine
     iii. repeated doses do not induce pharmacological tolerance
     iv. it is converted to an active metabolite
     v.   of its action as a bulk agent within the lumen of the bowel.

ASSERTION / REASON

9.32   Oral glucose electrolyte solutions are effective in the management of acute watery diarrhoea **BECAUSE** oral glucose electrolyte solutions are hypertonic.

9.33   The concomitant administration of antacid and cimetidine is not recommended **BECAUSE** cimetidine requires an acid environment in which to work.

9.34V   Alcohol ethoxylates (terics) act as antibloat agents in cattle **BECAUSE** alcohol ethoxylates hydrolyse saponins in the lumen.

ANSWERS

9.1	T	9.7	F	9.13	E	9.19	E	9.25	A	9.31	D
9.2	T	9.8	T	9.14	E	9.20	C	9.26	B	9.32	C
9.3	T	9.9	F	9.15	B	9.21	B	9.27	B	9.33	E
9.4	F	9.10	T	9.16	C	9.22	C	9.28	A	9.34	C
9.5	F	9.11	F	9.17	B	9.23	B	9.29	C		
9.6	F	9.12	T	9.18	B	9.24	C	9.30	A		

10 Drugs which Act on the Uterus

TRUE / FALSE

10.1 Oxytocin contracts smooth muscle in the mammary glands.

10.2 Ergometrine is a uterine stimulant which is excreted from the posterior pituitary.

10.3 The actions of ergometrine are more selectively oxytocic than those of dihydroergotamine.

10.4 Prostaglandin $F_{2\alpha}$ relaxes uterine smooth muscle.

10.5 Ergometrine is used therapeutically to enhance lactation when the suckling reflex is inadequate.

10.6 Sympathetic nervous activity causes strong rhythmic contractions of the uterus.

CORRECT OPTION

10.7 Which of the following organs, when stimulated, does not provoke the release of oxytocin?
    A. uterine cervix
    B. vagina
    C. breast
    D. oropharynx.

10.8 Ergometrine exerts its main effect on the :
    A. uterus
    B. peripheral nervous system
    C. kidney
    D. vascular system.

10.9 High levels of oestrogen markedly enhance the contractile response of uterine smooth muscle to:
    A. ergometrine
    B. oxytocin
    C. prostaglandin $F_{2\alpha}$
    D. salbutamol
    E. none of the above.

10.10   The treatment of choice for the induction of labour is:
      A.   oxytocin
      B.   adrenaline
      C.   prostaglandin E_2
      D.   ergometrine.

10.11   A.   In small doses, oxytocin has a direct relaxant effect on vascular smooth muscle in humans.
      B.   Vasopressin is twenty times more potent than oxytocin on uterine smooth muscle.
      C.   Oxytocin is the drug of choice for the induction of labour.
      D.   Oxytocin is not used to promote milk ejection.
      E.   Low blood levels of oestrogen increase the sensitivity of the uterus to oxytocin.

INCORRECT OPTION

10.12   In the lactating female, milk ejection is:
      A.   produced by oxytocin
      B.   produced by ethanol
      C.   produced in response to clitoral stimulation
      D.   not produced by ergotamine
      E.   inhibited by catecholamines.

10.13   Ergometrine is favoured over dihydroergotamine:
      A.   to treat postpartum haemorrhage
      B.   in the treatment of migraine
      C.   to promote uterine involution
      D.   to aid expulsion of the placenta.

10.14   Oxytocin:
      A.   causes contraction of myoepithelial cells in the mammary gland
      B.   increases the frequency of uterine contraction
      C.   in high doses, decreases blood pressure
      D.   increases the force of uterine contraction
      E.   causes maternal respiratory distress.

10.15   Oxytocin is effective when it is administered:
      A.   intravenously
      B.   intramuscularly
      C.   sublingually
      D.   orally
      E.   intranasally.

ASSERTION / REASON

10.16   For the induction of labour at full term, ergometrine is contraindicated **BECAUSE** ergometrine is likely to produce foetal hypoxia.

10.17   Vasopressin is used to induce labour **BECAUSE** vasopressin has a similar structure to oxytocin.

10.18   Ergometrine is preferred to oxytocin for the induction of labour **BECAUSE** ergometrine reduces the risk of post-partum haemorrhage.

10.19   Oxytocin is used to treat post-partum haemorrhage **BECAUSE** oxytocin produces contractions of the uterus.

ANSWERS

10.1 T	10.5 F	10.9 B	10.13 B	10.17 D
10.2 F	10.6 F	10.10 A	10.14 E	10.18 D
10.3 T	10.7 D	10.11 C	10.15 D	10.19 A
10.4 F	10.8 A	10.12 B	10.16 A	

11 Migraine

TRUE / FALSE

11.1   During an attack of migraine, blood levels of 5-hydroxytrytamine may fall by up to 80%.

11.2   Oral absorption of ergotamine is enhanced by caffeine.

11.3   β-Adrenoceptor antagonists are useful in some patients for migraine prophylaxis.

CORRECT OPTION

11.4   Which of the following drugs is not used in the prophylaxis of migraine?
   A.   dihydroergotamine
   B.   pizotifen
   C.   cyproheptadine
   D.   methysergide
   E.   clonidine.

11.5   Which of the following is not used in the management of migraine?
   A.   ergotamine
   B.   aspirin
   C.   metoclopramide
   D.   reserpine
   E.   methysergide.

INCORRECT OPTION

11.6   Acute attacks of migraine can be effectively treated with:
   A.   ergotamine
   B.   pethidine
   C.   aspirin plus metoclopramide
   D.   clonidine
   E.   dihydroergotamine.

MCQ

11.7   Current evidence suggests that the following may be involved in the pathogenesis of migraine:
     i.   5-hydroxytryptamine
     ii. γ-aminobutyric acid (GABA)
     iii. substance P
     iv. leukotrienes
     v.   oxygen free radicals.

11.8   An increased frequency of migraine headaches would be likely to occur as a result of:
     i.   commencement of a course of oral contraceptives
     ii.   ergotamine habituation
     iii. cessation of methysergide therapy
     iv. cessation of propranolol therapy.

ASSERTION / REASON

11.9.   Reserpine and fenfluramine may precipitate attacks of migraine **BECAUSE** reserpine and fenfluramine stimulate β-adrenoceptors.

11.10   The effectiveness of aspirin in the treatment of acute attacks of migraine is enhanced by metoclopramide **BECAUSE** metoclopramide has antinauseant actions.

ANSWERS

11.1 T	11.3 T	11.5 D	11.7 B	11.9 C
11.2 T	11.4 A	11.6 D	11.8 E	11.10 B

12 Hormones

12.1   Pituitary-derived β-endorphin is formed from the same precursor as corticotrophin.

12.2   The anterior pituitary gland controls the secretion of hormones by the adrenal cortex.

12.3   Drugs that block dopamine receptors may cause an elevation of plasma prolactin levels.

12.4   Some patients who take bromocriptine may develop galactorrhoea.

12.5   Ethanol stimulates the release of vasopressin.

12.6   Parathyroid hormone secretion is controlled by the hypothalamus and pituitary.

12.7   Both hypothyroidism and hyperthyroidism can be treated with iodide.

12.8V   Supplementary iodide is sometimes useful in the treatment of hypothyroidism.

12.9   Acute adrenal insufficiency may result from rapid withdrawal of corticosteroid therapy.

12.10   Prednisolone (40-50 mg/day) may produce Cushingoid symptoms.

12.11   Corticosteroids are useful as an initial single drug treatment for arthritis.

12.12   Metyrapone inhibits the synthesis of glucocorticoids but not that of mineralocorticoids.

12.13   Aldosterone deficiency results in excessive Na^+ loss.

12.14   Juvenile-onset diabetes is due to an absence of insulin in the pancreas.

12.15   Diet plays a very minor role in the treatment of diabetes.

12.16   Ultralente insulin is a complex of protamine, zinc and insulin.

12.17   Porcine insulin is generally less allergenic than bovine insulin.

12.18   Sulphonylureas may cause hypoglycaemia in non-diabetic individuals.

12.19   Sulphonylurea hypoglycaemics induce the release of insulin from pancreatic β-cells.

12.20   Sulphonylureas decrease the risk of coronary heart disease in diabetics.

12.21   Tolbutamide causes degranulation of the β-cells of the pancreas.

12.22   The oral hypoglycaemic actions of metformin are brought about by the stimulation of insulin release from the β-cells of the islets of Langerhans.

12.23   Biguanides interfere with glucose absorption.

12.24V Chorionic gonadotrophin is useful in cases of failure of lactation in sows and bitches.

12.25   Testosterone is effective if taken orally.

12.26   Androgens may produce remission in carcinoma of the prostate.

12.27   Testosterone may cause salt and water retention.

12.28   The retention of nitrogen induced by anabolic steroids is associated with increased protein synthesis.

12.29   Stanozolol is an effective anabolic agent.

12.30   Methyltestosterone may cause cholestatic jaundice.

12.31   Cyproterone is useful in the treatment of reduced libido in males.

12.32   The use of androgens in the treatment osteoporosis is associated with a decrease in bone resorption and improved Ca^{++} balance.

12.33V Large doses of androgens given to male animals may cause collapse and death within 48 hours.

12.34V Testosterone propionate will suppress oestrus in bitches.

12.35   Oestriol is the major secretory product of the ovary.

12.36   Oestrogens may alter blood clotting mechanisms.

12.37   Progesterone causes a decrease in body temperature.

12.38   Norethynodrel is a progestogen.

12.39   Clomiphene reduces gonadotrophin secretion.

12.40   Oestrogens may cause salt and water retention.

12.41   50 to 65% of all malignant breast tumours contain oestrogen receptors.

12.42V "Pregnant mare's serum" contains a mixture of oestrogens and progestogens.

CORRECT OPTION

12.43 Synthetic analogues of an endogenous hormone are used in replacement therapy for deficiency of:
    A.   thyroxine
    B.   aldosterone
    C.   gastrin
    D.   growth hormone
    E.   none of the above.

12.44 Which of the following is the agent of choice for the treatment of diabetes insipidus?
    A.   prednisolone
    B.   tolbutamide
    C.   ethanol
    D.   growth hormone
    E.   vasopressin.

12.45-12.48

12.45 somatostatin

12.46 growth hormone

12.47 vasopressin

12.48 aldosterone

For each of the compounds above, indicate whether it is secreted by the:

    A.   adrenal cortex
    B.   adenohypophysis
    C.   neurohypophysis
    D.   hypothalamus.

12.49-12.52

12.49 growth hormone

12.50 corticosteroids

12.51 antidiuretic hormone

12.52 insulin

For each of the hormones above, indicate whether it is appropriate therapy for:

    A.   diabetes insipidus
    B.   hypopituitary dwarfism
    C.   diabetes mellitus
    D.   osteoarthritis
    E.   infertility.

12.53   The actions of testosterone are inhibited by:
      A.   cyproterone
      B.   clomiphene
      C.   somatostatin
      D.   bromocriptine.

12.54   An example of a drug which acts by blocking endocrine hormone receptors in target cells is:
      A.   propylthiouracil
      B.   diazoxide
      C.   ornipressin
      D.   calcitonin
      E.   clomiphene.

12.55   Release of prolactin from the adenohypophysis is:
      A.   suppressed by somatostatin
      B.   suppressed by haloperidol
      C.   suppressed by bromocriptine
      D.   enhanced by dopamine
      E.   enhanced by oestradiol.

12.56   Corticotrophin:
      A.   is a glycoprotein
      B.   is effective in man only if derived from human sources
      C.   increases the release of aldosterone to a greater extent than that of hydrocortisone
      D.   release is increased by hydrocortisone
      E.   can be used as an anti-inflammatory agent.

12.57   Thyroxine and tri-iodothyronine are:
      A.   of similar potency
      B.   bound to plasma proteins to a similar extent
      C.   not absorbed when administered orally
      D.   inhibitors of thyrotrophin release
      E.   used to treat goitre in hyperthyroid patients.

12.58   Uptake of iodide into the thyroid gland is inhibited by:
      A.   propylthiouracil
      B.   iodine, in high doses
      C.   thyrotrophin
      D.   carbimazole
      E.   oestrogens.

12.59   Propylthiouracil is the preferred thionamide for the treatment of thyrotoxicosis because:
      A.   its plasma half-life is greater than 8 hours
      B.   it has a greater bioavailability than the other thionamides
      C.   it blocks iodine uptake by the thyroid gland
      D.   it inhibits peripheral conversion of thyroxine to tri-iodothyronine
      E.   none of the above.

12.60   In thyrotoxicosis, propranolol:
    A.   reduces the increased levels of circulating catecholamines
    B.   blocks the stimulating effects of autoantibodies on thyrotrophin receptors
    C.   abolishes the clinical manifestations of sympathetic overactivity
    D.   restores the ratio of thyroxine to tri-iodothyronine in plasma to normal
    E.   none of the above.

12.61   Corticotrophin is frequently used in the treatment of:
    A.   primary adrenal insufficiency
    B.   primary hypothyroidism
    C.   chronic asthma
    D.   pituitary insufficiency
    E.   none of the above.

12.62   Part of the anti-inflammatory effect of the corticosteroids is due to:
    A.   stimulation of renin release from the kidney
    B.   increased synthesis of insulin in the pancreas
    C.   inhibition of phospholipase A_2 activity
    D.   decreased production of bradykinin from plasma kininogen
    E.   decreased release of corticotrophin from the pituitary gland.

12.63   High doses of glucocorticoids can lead to all of the following symptoms except:
    A.   euphoria
    B.   increased skeletal muscle strength
    C.   moon face
    D.   hypertension
    E.   increased susceptibility to infection.

12.64   The steroid with the highest glucocorticoid/mineralocorticoid activity ratio is:
    A.   betamethasone
    B.   aldosterone
    C.   cortisone
    D.   fludrocortisone
    E.   prednisone.

12.65   The compound with the highest mineralocorticoid/glucocorticoid activity ratio is:
    A.   cortisone
    B.   betamethasone
    C.   prednisolone
    D.   fludrocortisone
    E.   deoxycorticosterone acetate.

12.66   Which of the following corticosteroids has the longest half-life?
    A.   hydrocortisone
    B.   cortisone
    C.   prednisolone
    D.   prednisone
    E.   dexamethasone.

Hormones

12.67 - 12.70

12.67   regular insulin

12.68   insulin zinc suspension (amorphous)

12.69   isophane insulin

12.70   lente insulin

For each of the formulations above, indicate the most likely pharmacokinetics:

	ONSET (min)	PEAK ACTIVITY (hrs)	DURATION OF ACTION (hrs)
A.	20-30	3-5	5-18
B.	30-45	4-6	12-18
C.	60-90	8-12	24-48.

12.71   Which of the following drugs may be useful in the treatment of maturity onset diabetes?
A.   glucose
B.   phenindione
C.   tolbutamide
D.   Δ-9-tetrahydrocannabinol
E.   propylthiouracil.

12.72   Which of the following drugs is not useful in the treatment of diabetes mellitus?
A.   glibenclamide
B.   isophane insulin
C.   chlorpropamide
D.   sulphamethazole
E.   metformin.

12.73   A similar duration of action is obtained with:
A.   insulin B.P. and insulin zinc suspension (crystalline) B.P.
B.   insulin zinc suspension (amorphous) B.P. and protamine zinc insulin B.P.
C.   protamine zinc insulin B.P. and isophane insulin B.P.
D.   isophane insulin B.P. and insulin zinc suspension B.P.
E.   insulin zinc suspension B.P. and insulin B.P.

12.74   Patients with mature-onset diabetes:
A.   usually rely heavily on insulin replacement therapy
B.   retain normal function in their islet β-cells
C.   do not respond to metformin
D.   may be treated with tolbutamide and dietary therapy
E.   may be subject to hypoglycaemic coma if untreated.

12.75V In dogs, one of the major side effects of tolbutamide is:
A.   nephrotoxicity
B.   cardiac failure
C.   hepatotoxicity
D.   pancreatitis
E.   none of the above.

12.76 Tolbutamide and metformin:
    A.   are sulphonylurea derivatives
    B.   release insulin from pancreatic β-cells
    C.   produce hypoglycaemia in normal subjects
    D.   may produce lactic acidosis
    E.   none of the above.

12.77 In patients being treated with anti-diabetic drugs, β-adrenoceptor antagonists must be used with caution because they:
    A.   enhance growth hormone secretion
    B.   suppress endogenous catecholamine-induced glycogenolysis
    C.   enhance endogenous catecholamine-induced glycogenolysis
    D.   antagonise the effects of biguanide-induced hyperglycaemia.

12.78 - 12.81

12.78V treatment of mammary tumours in bitches

12.79V increasing libido and sperm production in stallions

12.80V prevention of habitual abortion

12.81V prevention of pregnancy in bitches after misalliance

For each of the indications above, indicate the most appropriate hormone:

    A.   an androgen
    B.   an oestrogen
    C.   a progestogen
    D.   a gonadotrophin.

12.82 Which of the following steroids has no anabolic activity?
    A.   oxymetholone
    B.   fluoxymesterone
    C.   ethyloestrenol
    D.   nandrolone esters
    E.   megestrol.

12.83 Which of the following has anabolic actions without appreciable androgenic side effects?
    A.   methyltestosterone
    B.   methandriol
    C.   nandrolone
    D.   norethisterone
    E.   none of the above.

Hormones

12.84 - 12.88

12.84   tamoxifen

12.85   17-α-ethinyloestrenol

12.86   17-α-ethinyloestradiol

12.87   testosterone

12.88   nortestosterone

For each of the compounds listed above, indicate whether it is:

A.   a progestogen
B.   an oestrogen
C.   an androgen
D.   an anabolic steroid
E.   an antioestrogen.

12.89   Which of the following is not an indication for the use of progestational agents?
A.   contraception
B.   dysmenorrhoea
C.   stimulation of postpartum lactation
D.   threatened or habitual abortion
E.   dysfunctional uterine bleeding.

12.90   All oral contraceptive preparations:
A.   contain oestrogen
B.   have a 5% failure rate
C.   are commonly associated with infertility after withdrawal
D.   alter the characteristics of the cervical mucus
E.   act principally by inhibiting ovulation.

12.91   Which of the following hormonal effects is unlikely to contribute to oral contraceptive efficacy?
A.   an elevation of luteinising hormone
B.   inhibition of ovulation
C.   change in the quality and quantity of cervical mucus
D.   an abnormal proliferative and/or secretory endometrial phase
E.   inhibition of nidation.

12.92   Which of the following side effects is least likely with the use of oral contraceptives?
A.   migraine
B.   kidney disease
C.   breast fullness
D.   oedema and weight gain
E.   nausea.

INCORRECT OPTION

12.93 Endogenous hormones which are used therapeutically or diagnostically include:
    A. growth hormone
    B. prolactin
    C. parathyroid hormone
    D. calcitonin
    E. glucagon.

12.94 Somatomedins:
    A. stimulate protein growth in bone and muscle
    B. are active both *in vivo* and *in vitro*
    C. have a steroid nucleus
    D. inhibit the release of growth hormone
    E. are not anterior pituitary hormones.

12.95 Glucocorticoids:
    A. produce hyperglycaemia
    B. produce immunosuppression
    C. suppress corticotrophin release
    D. may suppress prostaglandin synthesis
    E. increase the growth of lymphoid tissue.

12.96 The iodination and coupling steps in the biosynthesis of thyroxine and tri-iodothyronine are impaired by:
    A. propylthiouracil
    B. iodine in high doses
    C. thiocyanates
    D. carbimazole
    E. methimazole.

12.97 Actions of testosterone at puberty include:
    A. growth of body and facial hair
    B. development of skeletal muscle
    C. increased subcutaneous fat
    D. laryngeal growth
    E. increased secretions from sebaceous glands.

12.98 Oestrogens are useful in:
    A. oral contraception
    B. endometriosis
    C. dysmenorrhoea
    D. post-menopausal hormone replacement therapy
    E. osteoporosis.

12.99 Ethinyloestradiol:
    A. suppresses the release of follicle-stimulating hormone
    B. can initiate oestrus
    C. can suppress ovulation
    D. can prevent nidation
    E. is ineffective when administered orally.

12.100V Oestrogens may be used to:
    A.   induce ovulation in mares
    B.   induce oestrus in sheep
    C.   reduce excessive libido in male dogs
    D.   reduce mammary tumours in bitches
    E.   reduce urinary incontinence in spayed bitches.

MCQ

12.101 Somatomedins:
    i.   inhibit the release of growth hormone
    ii.   enhance the release of growth hormone
    iii.   mediate many of the actions of growth hormone
    iv.   inhibit the release of somatostatin
    v.   enhance the release of somatostatin.

12.102 Which of the following statements is/are true?
    i.   Propylthiouracil inhibits oxidation of iodide to iodine and its coupling to tyrosine.
    ii.   Tolbutamide may cause anaerobic glycolysis.
    iii.   Semilente insulin is a relatively short acting insulin.
    iv.   Protamine zinc insulin should, on theoretical grounds, have fewer side effects than "regular" insulin.
    v.   Heat intolerance is a key feature of hypothyroidism.

12.103 Anti-diuretic hormone:
    i.   releases vasoactive intestinal peptide
    ii.   release is inhibited by ethanol
    iii.   is released in response to a decrease in plasma osmotic pressure
    iv.   causes vasoconstriction at high doses
    v.   causes contraction of the uterus during labour.

12.104 Follicle-stimulating hormone:
    i.   is an anterior pituitary hormone
    ii.   stimulates testosterone secretion in the testis
    iii.   stimulates oestradiol secretion in the ovary
    iv.   enhances the release of luteinising hormone
    v.   enhances the release of prolactin.

12.105 Carbimazole:
    i.   is useful in the treatment of hyperthyroidism
    ii.   is 10 times more potent than methimazole
    iii.   may rarely cause agranulocytosis
    iv.   is less toxic than propylthiouracil
    v.   must be given by injection.

12.106 The antithyroid action of propylthiouracil involves:
    i.   suppression of the conversion of thyroxine to tri-iodothyronine in peripheral tissues
    ii.   suppression of the coupling reactions in the biosynthesis of thyroid hormones
    iii.   suppression of the iodination reactions in the biosynthesis of thyroid hormones
    iv.   suppression of iodine uptake into the thyroid gland cell
    v.   its prior conversion to thiouracil.

12.107 Which of the following are clinically effective as topical preparations?
    i.   cortisone
    ii.   hydrocortisone
    iii. prednisone
    iv.   prednisolone
    v.   adrenocorticotrophic hormone.

12.108 The short-term effects of systemic treatment with high doses of corticosteroids are:
    i.   hypertension
    ii.   mood changes
    iii. osteoporosis
    iv.   hypokalaemia
    v.   Cushing's syndrome.

12.109 Side effects of chlorpropamide include:
    i.   ethanol intolerance
    ii.   weight gain
    iii. hypoglycaemia
    iv.   fluid retention
    v.   skin rashes.

12.110 Osteoporosis:
    i.   occurs in hypercortisolism
    ii.   may be due to the administration of anti-inflammatory steroids
    iii. is associated with increased urinary excretion of hydroxyproline
    iv.   is more common in patients who have had oophorectomies
    v.   in menopausal women can be treated successfully with oestrogens and calcium gluconate.

12.111 Oestrogens:
    i.   are one of the constituents of the "mini-pill"
    ii.   in large doses are used for post-coital contraception
    iii. all have a steroidal structure
    iv.   are useful in the treatment of menopausal symptoms
    v.   are incorporated into intrauterine contraceptive devices.

12.112 Which of the following statements is/are true?
    i.   Progesterone is the main hormone sustaining the secretory phase of endometrial proliferation during the menstrual cycle.
    ii.   Clomiphene induces ovulation because it is structurally similar to follicle-stimulating hormone.
    iii. Synthetic progestins are the main constituents of the "mini-pill".
    iv.   Human chorionic gonadotrophin is extracted in large quantities from the urine of post-menopausal women.

12.113 Progestins:
    i.   suppress the release of hypothalamic gonadotrophin-releasing hormone
    ii.   suppress the release of chorionic gonadotrophin
    iii. suppress the release of luteinising hormone
    iv.   enhance the release of follicle-stimulating hormone
    v.   enhance the release of prolactin.

ASSERTION / REASON

12.114 Bromocriptine is useful in the treatment of infertility **BECAUSE** the dopamine-like activity of bromocriptine suppresses prolactin release.

12.115 Lysine-8-vasopressin can be used in patients who are allergic to animal vasopressin **BECAUSE** lysine-8-vasopressin is extracted from human plasma.

12.116 Thyrotrophin is used in the treatment of hypothyroidism **BECAUSE** thyrotrophin stimulates the synthesis and release of thyroxine and tri-iodothyronine.

12.117 Orally administered insulin does not produce hypoglycaemia in non-diabetic people **BECAUSE** in non-diabetic people, blood glucose levels influence the release of insulin from the β-cells of the pancreas.

12.118 Sulphonylurea drugs are the treatment of choice for obese type 2 diabetics **BECAUSE** sulphonylurea drugs cause weight loss.

12.119 Osteoporosis can be caused by androgens **BECAUSE** androgens chelate calcium ions.

12.120 Anabolic steroids are useful in the treatment of cancer of the prostate **BECAUSE** anabolic steroids all have some androgenic activity.

12.121 The use of anabolic steroids to improve performance in athletes is undesirable **BECAUSE** anabolic steroids are not absorbed after oral administration.

12.122 Diethylstilboestrol is a potent oestrogenic compound **BECAUSE** diethylstilboestrol has a steroid structure similar to that of oestrogen.

12.123V Large doses of stilboestrol can induce abortion if administered within 48 hours of mating **BECAUSE** stilboestrol has potent antioestrogenic activity.

12.124 Oral contraceptive hormones are potentially dangerous in women of 35 years and over who smoke **BECAUSE** oral contraceptive hormones greatly increase the risk of thrombotic disorders in women of 35 years and over who smoke.

12.125V Progesterone is a useful contraceptive in bitches **BECAUSE** progesterone reduces follicle-stimulating hormone and luteinising hormone release from the pituitary.

ANSWERS

12.1	T	12.26	F	12.51	A	12.76	D	12.101	B
12.2	T	12.27	T	12.52	C	12.77	B	12.102	B
12.3	T	12.28	T	12.53	A	12.78	A	12.103	C
12.4	F	12.29	T	12.54	E	12.79	D	12.104	B
12.5	F	12.30	T	12.55	C	12.80	C	12.105	B
12.6	F	12.31	F	12.56	E	12.81	B	12.106	A
12.7	T	12.32	T	12.57	D	12.82	E	12.107	C
12.8	T	12.33	F	12.58	B	12.83	C	12.108	E
12.9	T	12.34	T	12.59	D	12.84	E	12.109	E
12.10	T	12.35	F	12.60	C	12.85	A	12.110	E
12.11	F	12.36	T	12.61	D	12.86	B	12.111	D
12.12	T	12.37	F	12.62	C	12.87	C	12.112	B
12.13	T	12.38	T	12.63	B	12.88	D	12.113	B
12.14	T	12.39	F	12.64	A	12.89	C	12.114	A
12.15	F	12.40	T	12.65	D	12.90	D	12.115	C
12.16	F	12.41	T	12.66	E	12.91	A	12.116	D
12.17	T	12.42	F	12.67	A	12.92	B	12.117	B
12.18	T	12.43	B	12.68	A	12.93	B	12.118	E
12.19	T	12.44	E	12.69	B	12.94	C	12.119	C
12.20	F	12.45	D	12.70	C	12.95	E	12.120	D
12.21	T	12.46	B	12.71	C	12.96	C	12.121	C
12.22	F	12.47	C	12.72	D	12.97	C	12.122	C
12.23	T	12.48	A	12.73	D	12.98	B	12.123	C
12.24	T	12.49	B	12.74	D	12.99	E	12.124	A
12.25	F	12.50	D	12.75	C	12.100	D	12.125	A

13 Vitamins

TRUE / FALSE

13.1   In order to maintain normal health, it is necessary that vitamin intake be on a daily basis.

13.2   Administration of a therapeutic dose of a vitamin will have no effect unless there is a prior deficiency.

13.3   A majority of the water soluble vitamins can be synthesised by normal intestinal flora.

13.4   Vitamin A is stored in the liver as esters of long chain aliphatic acids.

13.5   Most vitamins of the B complex have been shown to be components of enzyme systems.

13.6V   Chickens possess enzymes to synthesise their own vitamin B_1.

13.7V   In most farm animals, a majority of the B group vitamins are synthesised by intestinal flora.

13.8   A vitamin C-free diet for 2 weeks will cause body stores of vitamin C to fall to less than 5% of normal.

13.9V   Dogs do not normally require an exogenous source of vitamin C for normal health.

13.10   Vitamin D_3 (cholecalciferol) is the biologically active form of the vitamin which increases calcium absorption from the gut and renal tubules.

13.11   Vitamin E deficiency causes muscular dystrophy.

13.12   Vitamin E can be used to treat warfarin poisoning.

13.13   Topical use of vitamin K and a related acid is helpful in the treatment of acne.

CORRECT OPTION

13.14   Vitamin C:
    A.   deficiency leads to beri-beri
    B.   deficiency is apparent in 30% of the Australian population
    C.   is lost from the body at the rate of 3-4% of the total body store per day
    D.   is stable to heat
    E.   derivatives are used topically to treat certain types of acne.

13.15 - 13.16

13.15   folic acid

13.16   vitamin K

For each of the substances above, indicate whether its actions are mimicked or antagonised by:

    A.   sulphadimidine
    B.   mepyramine
    C.   methotrexate
    D.   warfarin.

13.17 - 13.18

13.17   beri-beri

13.18   pellagra

For each of the vitamin deficiency syndromes above, the best treatment is:

    A.   thiamine
    B.   riboflavine
    C.   nicotinic acid
    D.   pyridoxine
    E.   ascorbic acid.

INCORRECT OPTION

13.19   Vitamin deficiency:
    A.   is best treated by doses of the appropriate vitamin
    B.   commonly results from unbalanced diets
    C.   symptoms generally appear within a month of dietary deprivation
    D.   syndromes are easy to relate to particular enzyme systems involved.

13.20 Ascorbic acid:
    A.   is rapidly absorbed from the intestinal tract
    B.   plasma levels can become low on abrupt cessation of a very high vitamin C diet
    C.   is utilised at an increased rate during infection
    D.   is reversibly oxidised to oxalic acid
    E.   protects against scurvy at a dose of 10 mg/day.

13.21 Vitamin D:
    A.   is useful in the treatment of hyperthyroidism
    B.   can be toxic in high doses
    C.   deficiency frequently results in rickets in children
    D.   intake is not normally needed if a person gets sufficient sunlight
    E.   absorption from the gastrointestinal tract is decreased in the presence of large amounts of liquid paraffin.

13.22 Vitamin D:
    A.   is a fat soluble vitamin
    B.   is inactivated by sunlight
    C.   is a steroid-derived vitamin
    D.   can cause toxic effects in overdose
    E.   causes increased absorption of dietary calcium.

13.23 Vitamin E:
    A.   acts as a fat soluble anti-oxidant
    B.   deficiency occurs rarely, if at all, in adult man
    C.   has been proved essential for reproduction in man
    D.   includes α-tocopherol
    E.   occurs in nuts.

13.24V Vitamin E:
    A.   is not essential for reproduction in most animal species
    B.   deficiency may be treated with a high dietary intake of unsaturated fats
    C.   deficiencies are rare in adult animals
    D.   acts as an anti-oxidant
    E.   and selenium treatment is effective for white muscle disease in calves.

MCQ

13.25 Vitamin D_3 (cholecalciferol):
    i.   is effective treatment for osteomalacia
    ii.   increases calcium reabsorption from the renal tubule
    iii.   facilitates the absorption of calcium from the intestine
    iv.   is inactivated in the liver by conversion to 1,25-dihydroxy-D_3
    v.   stimulates the release of parathyroid hormone from the parathyroid gland.

13.26   Which of the following are active as antiscorbutic agents?
       i.   ascorbic acid
      ii.   oxalic acid
    iii. dehydroascorbic acid
    iv. vitamin E
     v.   glucose.

13.27   The use of .... may necessitate supplementary vitamin therapy with
        .... Which of the following correctly completes the sentence?
       i.   antibiotics such as tetracyclines;   vitamin E
      ii.   ethanol;   vitamin A
    iii. tryptophan;   nicotinamide
    iv. oral contraceptives;   pyridoxine.

ANSWERS

13.1	F	13.7	T	13.13	F	13.19	C	13.25	A
13.2	T	13.8	F	13.14	C	13.20	D	13.26	B
13.3	T	13.9	T	13.15	C	13.21	A	13.27	D
13.4	T	13.10	F	13.16	D	13.22	B		
13.5	T	13.11	T	13.17	A	13.23	C		
13.6	F	13.12	F	13.18	C	13.24	B		

14 Chemotherapy

TRUE / FALSE

14.1   Superinfection is an overwhelming invasion of pathogens.

14.2   Antibiotics always originate from moulds.

14.3   Disinfectants are bactericidal.

14.4   To be effective, antibiotics must be bactericidal.

14.5   There is always a direct relationship between the minimum inhibitory concentrations of antibiotics in bacterial cultures and the efficacy of the antibiotics *in vivo*.

14.6   The development of safe and effective antibacterial drugs has made it unnecessary to drain surgical wounds.

14.7   If two bacteriostatic drugs are used together, a bactericidal effect often results.

In antibacterial treatment it is correct and justifiable:

14.8   to combine any two or more antibiotics.

14.9   to combine penicillin with streptomycin.

14.10   to combine oxytetracycline and chloramphenicol.

14.11   to give slowly increasing doses of antibiotics.

14.12   to achieve and to maintain therapeutically effective blood concentrations of antibiotics as quickly as possible.

14.13   R-factor transfer can confer multiple drug resistance on an organism.

14.14   Resistance to tetracyclines may occur by R-factor transfer of genes which increase the rate of destruction of the drug.

14.15   Genetic material conferring multiple antibiotic resistance can be transferred from commensal organisms to pathogens.

14.16   Bacterial resistance to chemotherapeutic drugs can eventually be overcome by prolonged low-dose therapy.

14.17 Pyrimethamine and proguanil are the drugs of choice to terminate an acute attack of malaria.

14.18 The antimalarial action of proguanil involves inhibition of dihydrofolate reductase.

14.19 The principal use of primaquine is for the radical curative treatment of *vivax* malaria.

14.20 Patients must always be purged after taking taenicides.

14.21V The most important reason for treating nematode infestations in domestic animals is to minimise risks to human health.

14.22 Piperazine is poorly absorbed from the gastrointestinal tract.

14.23 Piperazine acts by inhibiting carbohydrate metabolism in roundworms.

14.24 Pyrantel pamoate antagonises the effects of piperazine on parasitic worms.

14.25 The mechanism of action of niclosamide in the chemotherapy of tapeworm infestation precludes the development of cysticercosis in *Taenia solium* infestation.

14.26 Niclosamide kills both the worm and viable eggs.

14.27 Niclosamide is not extensively absorbed from the gastrointestinal tract.

14.28 Diloxanide effectively eliminates *Entamoeba histolytica* from the liver.

14.29 Metronidazole inhibits aldehyde dehydrogenase.

14.30V Amprolium acts as a folic acid antagonist in controlling coccidiosis in poultry.

14.31 p-Aminobenzoic acid inhibits the antibacterial action of sulphonamides.

14.32 Bacterial resistance to sulphonamides can occur by R-factor transfer.

14.33 Alkalinisation of the urine is necessary when sulphamethizole is administered.

14.34 Methicillin is resistant to destruction by gastric acid.

14.35 Methicillin is resistant to staphylococcal penicillinases.

14.36 In the treatment of severely ill patients, procaine penicillin can be given by intravenous injection.

14.37 Oral phenoxymethylpenicillin is a suitable treatment for life-threatening infections due to sensitive organisms.

14.38 Amoxycillin is a β-lactam antibiotic with good acid stability.

14.39 Amoxycillin readily crosses the blood-brain barrier.

14.40   The half-life of amoxycillin is significantly increased in elderly women with normal blood urea and serum creatinine levels.

14.41   The presence of food in the stomach delays and reduces the absorption of amoxycillin.

14.42   The pharmacokinetics of amoxycillin and potassium clavulanate are similar.

14.43   Synergistic effects between penicillin and chloramphenicol may occur.

14.44   The fixed combination of trimethoprim and sulphamethoxazole can be used interchangeably with penicillin.

14.45   Azlocillin has synergistic activity with gentamicin and sisomycin.

14.46   Although inactivated by most β-lactamases, piperacillin is active against some strains of β-lactamase producing gonococci.

14.47   There is no significant prolongation of the serum half-life of piperacillin in patients with impaired renal function.

14.48   Nafcillin is a potent, penicillinase-resistant penicillin.

14.49   Carbenicillin has activity against gram-negative organisms such as *Pseudomonas* species.

14.50   The antibacterial activity of carindacillin is entirely due to its conversion to carbenicillin.

14.51   In the presence of mecillinam, morphological changes occur in sensitive bacteria which render them very sensitive to the actions of penicillins and cephalosporins.

14.52   The high bactericidal activity of imipenem appears to relate to the rapid penetration of the drug into bacterial cells and an enhanced affinity for target sites responsible for cell wall synthesis.

14.53   Ticarcillin is stable in the presence of penicillinase.

14.54   The use of ticarcillin has led to the development of psuedomembranous colitis as a result of colonisation with *Clostridium difficile*, a toxin-producing organism.

14.55   Oral therapy with ampicillin is effective in the treatment of serious infections of the central nervous system.

14.56   The total free antibiotic levels achieved after oral administration of flucloxacillin are lower than those reached after the same dose of cloxacillin.

14.57   Pivampicillin is a pro-drug.

14.58   Penicillinase-producing organisms are resistant to cephalosporins.

14.59   Cefoxitin is stable to β-lactamases.

14.60 Cefuroxime axetil has almost no intrinsic antibacterial activity but is de-esterified by intestinal enzymes to produce cefuroxime.

14.61 The α-methoxamino substituent at position 7 on the β-lactam ring of ceftriaxone provides stability against β-lactamase.

14.62 Cefaclor is chemically and pharmacologically similar to cephalexin.

14.63 Methicillin-resistant staphyloccoci are almost uniformly sensitive to cefoxitin.

14.64 Cefoxitin is readily absorbed after oral administration.

14.65 Concomitant administration of probenecid decreases the renal clearance of cefoxitin.

14.66 Cefotaxime is a third generation cephalosporin which is resistant to several β-lactamases of gram negative bacilli.

14.67 Cephamandole has an attenuated "antabuse"-like interaction with ethanol.

14.68 Cross-resistance among aminoglycoside antibiotics is uncommon.

14.69 Aminoglycoside antibiotics have neuromuscular blocking activity.

14.70 Synergistic effects may occur between streptomycin and tetracycline.

14.71 In renal failure, gentamicin dosage is adjusted according to the creatinine clearance.

14.72 Tobramycin is more toxic than gentamicin.

14.73 Gentamicin is excreted almost entirely by renal glomerular filtration.

14.74 Congestive cardiac failure may alter the pharmacokinetics of gentamicin in the elderly patients.

14.75 Amikacin is an analogue of kanamycin.

14.76 Netilmicin inhibits protein synthesis in susceptible bacteria.

14.77 In patients with impaired renal function, the half-life of netilmicin decreases proportionally with the decrease in creatinine clearance.

14.78 The selective toxicity of tetracyclines depends on differential rates of entry into bacterial and mammalian cells.

14.79 Tetracycline may be inactivated by divalent and trivalent cations.

14.80 All tetracyclines are potentially hepatotoxic in pregnancy.

14.81 To prevent gastrointestinal irritation, tetracyclines should be administered with milk or antacids.

14.82 Doxycycline has a considerably longer duration of action than tetracycline.

14.83 Doxycycline is excreted mainly in the urine.

14.84 Erythromycin and chloramphenicol have synergistic effects.

14.85 Bone marrow depression has never been recorded following the topical use of chloramphenicol eye drops.

14.86 The polyene antifungal agents (e.g. nystatin) act by affecting the permeability of the cell membrane.

14.87 Nystatin-tetracycline combinations given by mouth prevent the occurrence of vaginal candidiasis.

14.88 Idoxuridine is preferred to cytarabine for the treatment of *Herpes simplex* encephalitis.

14.89 Trimethoprim is a competitive inhibitor of dihydrofolate reductase.

14.90 Erythromycin is concentrated many-fold in the bile.

14.91 Antibiotic anti-cancer drugs prevent bacterial infection in neutropaenic patients.

14.92 Cyclophosphamide forms an active metabolite.

14.93 Methotrexate inhibits the incorporation of folic acid into DNA.

CORRECT OPTION

14.94 Chemotherapy may be defined as:
    A.   the use of chemical substances to destroy infecting organisms
    B.   the use of drugs to injure invading organisms without injuring the host
    C.   the topical use of antiseptics
    D.   the use of antibiotics to provide cover against invading organisms
    E.   the use of antibiotics to injure bacteria.

14.95 The ideal chemotherapeutic agent has all of the following properties except:
    A.   selective and effective antimicrobial activity
    B.   bacteriostatic rather than bactericidal activity
    C.   does not induce resistance
    D.   maintains its antimicrobial activity in the presence of fluids, exudates, enzymes and plasma proteins
    E.   achieves and maintains therapeutic levels in blood and tissues.

14.96 Drug resistance in bacteria does not involve:
    A.   production of antibiotic-degrading enzymes
    B.   production of an essential metabolite
    C.   morphological alterations which restrict the entry of the antibiotic into the cell.
    D.   altered metabolic pathways
    E.   transfer of extra-chromosomal protein resistance factors.

14.97 - 14.98

14.97   phenoxymethylpenicillin

14.98   sulphadiazine

For each of the drugs above indicate whether it acts by:

A.   inhibition of cell wall synthesis
B.   inhibition of nucleic acid synthesis by reduced production of tetrahydrofolate
C.   inhibition of nucleic acid synthesis by competition with purines or pyrimidines
D.   inhibition of nucleic acid synthesis by combining with nucleic acid.

14.99 - 14.101

14.99   tetracycline

14.100   benzylpenicillin

14.101   colistin

For each of the drugs above, indicate whether it:

A.   blocks cross-linking in the bacterial cell wall
B.   is an antimetabolite
C.   is a bactericidal inhibitor of bacterial protein synthesis
D.   is a bacteriostatic inhibitor of bacterial protein synthesis
E.   affects the barrier function of the bacterial cell membrane.

14.102 - 14.105

14.102   cephaloridine

14.103   nystatin

14.104   erythromycin

14.105   streptomycin

For each of the drugs above, indicate whether it:

A.   causes the ribosome to miscode, with resultant aberrant protein synthesis
B.   acts on the early stages of protein manufacture by inhibition of ribosomal peptidyl transferase
C.   affects the barrier function of the cell membrane
D.   affects DNA replication in the chromosome
E.   inhibits bacterial cell wall synthesis.

14.106   Which of the following is not an accepted form of treatment for acute
         urinary tract infection?
         A.   co-trimoxazole for 5 days
         B.   phenoxymethylpenicillin - single dose
         C.   kanamycin - single i.m. dose
         D.   amoxycillin for 5-7 days
         E.   sulphafurazole for 7 days.

14.107   Which of the following antibiotics is bacteriostatic?
         A.   chloramphenicol
         B.   cephaloridine
         C.   cloxacillin
         D.   gentamicin
         E.   carbenicillin.

14.108   The antimalarial action of pyrimethamine is due to its ability to:
         A.   inhibit the incorporation of p-aminobenzoic acid into folic acid
         B.   immobilise   the   sporozoites   before   they   can   enter
              reticulo-endothelial cells
         C.   inhibit dihydrofolate reductase
         D.   cross-link the double DNA strands in the parasite
         E.   stimulate the defence mechanisms in the body so that partial
              immunity to malaria develops.

14.109   Primaquine causes haemolytic anaemia because one of its metabolites:
         A.   inhibits dihydrofolate reductase
         B.   inhibits glucose-6-phosphate dehydrogenase
         C.   oxidises glutathione
         D.   interferes with lipoprotein synthesis
         E.   produces methaemoglobinaemia.

14.110   A lethal effect on the exo-erythrocyte stage of *Plasmodium vivax* is
         produced by:
         A.   chloroquine
         B.   primaquine
         C.   quinine
         D.   proguanil
         E.   pyrimethamine.

14.111   Human infestation with *Trichinella spiralis* is readily controlled by:
         A.   pyrantel
         B.   piperazine
         C.   niclosamide
         D.   niridazole
         E.   none of the above

Chemotherapy

14.112 -14.115

14.112 niclosamide

14.113 viprynium

14.114 bephenium

14.115 niridazole

For each of the anthelmintics above, indicate whether it is most effective in the treatment of:

A. *Taenia saginata* (beef tapeworm)
B. *Schistosoma haematobium* (liver fluke)
C. *Enterobius (oxyuris) vermicularis* (pinworm)
D. *Ancylostoma duodenale* (hookworm).

14.116 - 14.120

14.116V effective against most nematode infestations, its mode of action involving inhibition of glucose uptake

14.117V has an anti-ascarid action, involving hyperpolarisation and consequent paralysis of the parasite

14.118V has a similar spectrum of anthelmintic efficacy to niclosamide

14.119V is effective in the treatment of *Fasciola hepatica* infestations

14.120V acts as an anthelmintic by means of an anticholinesterase action

For each of the descriptions above, indicate whether it applies to:

A. levamisole
B. mebendazole
C. nitroxynil
D. pyrantel
E. none of the above.

14.121 Metronidazole:
A. can only be used in the intra-intestinal form of amoebiasis
B. can only be used in the extra-intestinal form of amoebiasis
C. is of no use in the treatment of the carrier state
D. although effective, is reserved for serious cases because of its high toxicity
E. has its amoebicidal action reduced by ethanolic beverages.

14.122 The Wood-Fildes hypothesis of the antibacterial action of the sulphonamides is concerned with:
A. utilisation of amino acids
B. inhibition of respiration
C. folic acid synthesis
D. p-aminobenzoic acid synthesis
E. misreading of the genetic code.

14.123　Which of the following synthetic drugs mimics or antagonises the action of the natural substance p-aminobenzoic acid?
　　　A.　sulphadimidine
　　　B.　mepyramine
　　　C.　methotrexate
　　　D.　warfarin.

14.124　For the prevention of burn sepsis, the most useful drug is:
　　　A.　sulphamethizole
　　　B.　sulphasalazine
　　　C.　silver sulphadiazine
　　　D.　succinylsulphathiazole
　　　E.　sulphacetamide.

14.125　The drug of choice for treating *Haemophilis influenzae* meningitis is:
　　　A.　chloramphenicol
　　　B.　benzylpenicillin
　　　C.　lincomycin
　　　D.　erythromycin
　　　E.　amphotericin-B.

14.126　For patients who are allergic to penicillin, the most suitable antibiotic for the treatment of systemic infections would be:
　　　A.　cloxacillin
　　　B.　streptomycin
　　　C.　chloramphenicol
　　　D.　erythromycin
　　　E.　phenoxymethylpenicillin.

14.127　The most effective penicillin for the treatment of *Pseudomonas* infections is:
　　　A.　amoxycillin
　　　B.　benzylpenicillin
　　　C.　carbenicillin
　　　D.　procaine penicillin
　　　E.　epicillin.

14.128　An effective blood level of penicillin may be reached promptly by:
　　　A.　an oral dose of phenoxymethylpenicillin
　　　B.　an intramuscular injection of procaine penicillin
　　　C.　an intramuscular injection of benzylpenicillin
　　　D.　an intravenous injection of benzathine penicillin
　　　E.　an intravenous injection of procaine penicillin.

14.129　Benzylpenicillin:
　　　A.　is stable in acidic gastric contents
　　　B.　is resistant to staphylococcal penicillinase
　　　C.　readily crosses the blood-brain barrier when the meninges are normal
　　　D.　reaches high concentrations in ocular fluids
　　　E.　reaches high concentrations in proximal renal tubular cells.

14.130 - 14.132

14.130 procaine penicillin

14.131 flucloxacillin

14.132 amoxycillin

For each of the drugs above, indicate whether it:

    A.   has only very weak antibacterial activity
    B.   has activity against gram-negative organisms
    C.   acts as a depot after intramuscular administration
    D.   should be reserved for severe infections by penicillinase-producing organisms.

14.133 Tetracyclines:
    A.   are not absorbed from the gastrointestinal tract
    B.   are incompletely absorbed from the gastrointestinal tract
    C.   are better absorbed from the gastrointestinal tract when the patient is also taking certain antacid preparations
    D.   undergo hepatic recycling.

14.134 The use of chloramphenicol may be associated with the development of:
    A.   allergic rash
    B.   blood dyscrasias
    C.   sedation
    D.   alopecia
    E.   hepatotoxicity.

14.135 Acyclovir is ineffective against:
    A.   *Herpes simplex* type 1
    B.   *Varicella zoster*
    C.   *Herpes simplex* type 2
    D.   *Vaccinia*
    E.   Epstein-Barr virus.

14.136 Fungal infection of the skin produced by *Trichophyton* species can be treated effectively with:
    A.   topically applied griseofulvin
    B.   topically applied nystatin
    C.   topically applied miconazole
    D.   orally administered metronidazole
    E.   orally administered tolnaftate.

14.137 Nystatin acts by:
    A.   inhibition of protein synthesis by prevention of ribosomal binding of amino acyl-t-RNA
    B.   inhibition of protein synthesis by inhibition of ribosomal peptidyl transferase
    C.   inhibition of protein synthesis by blocking the translocation step
    D.   primary damage to cell membranes.

14.138 Which of the following antifungal agents is effective in both tinea and candidiasis?
    A.   nystatin
    B.   tolnaftate
    C.   miconazole
    D.   fluorocytosine
    E.   undecenoic acid.

14.139 The drug of choice for systemic infections by *Aspergillus fumigatus* is:
    A.   griseofulvin
    B.   idoxuridine
    C.   nystatin
    D.   amphotericin-B
    E.   none of the above.

14.140 Polymyxin B:
    A.   affects cell wall synthesis
    B.   inhibits protein synthesis
    C.   inhibits nucleic acid synthesis
    D.   acts as an antimetabolite
    E.   affects cell membrane permeability.

14.141 Which combination of cancer chemotherapeutic drugs would you expect to be most effective?
    A.   vincristine + doxorubicin
    B.   cyclophosphamide + methotrexate
    C.   cyclophosphamide + mustine
    D.   fluorouracil + cytarabine.

14.142 Antibiotic anti-cancer drugs:
    A.   intercalate and bind to DNA
    B.   are useful in cancer patients with infection
    C.   are mitotic spindle poisons
    D.   are specific enzyme inhibitors.

14.143 Alkylating agents kill tumour cells:
    A.   by arresting cells at metaphases
    B.   by reacting with nucleophilic DNA bases in tumour cells
    C.   by total inhibition of DNA/RNA polymerases
    D.   by reducing systemic L-asparaginase levels
    E.   only after hepatic microsomal activation of the drug

14.144 Methotrexate specifically inhibits:
    A.   hypoxanthine-guanine phosphoribosyltransferase
    B.   DNA polymerase
    C.   dihydrofolate reductase
    D.   thymidylate synthetase.

14.145 Methotrexate is used in cancer chemotherapy because:
    A.   it is harmless to all mammals
    B.   it is essential to cell reproduction
    C.   it structurally resembles folic acid
    D.   it attacks DNA molecules.

14.146 The predominant toxicity seen with vincristine therapy is:
  A. haemorrhagic cystitis
  B. nephrotoxicity
  C. neutropaenia
  D. peripheral neuropathy.

14.147 Vincristine is an:
  A. antibiotic
  B. alkylating agent
  C. antimetabolite
  D. alkaloid.

14.148 Methotrexate is:
  A. an antibiotic
  B. a pyrimidine base analogue
  C. an antimetabolite
  D. a DNA intercalating drug
  E. a mitotic spindle poison

INCORRECT OPTION

14.149 Resistance tends to develop when antibiotic use is:
  A. intermittent
  B. in too low a dose
  C. initiated early in infection
  D. of brief duration.

14.150 The antimalarial agent chloroquine:
  A. is effective in the treatment of giardiasis
  B. is effective in the treatment of extra-intestinal amoebiasis
  C. is effective in the treatment of toxoplasmosis
  D. has anti-inflammatory activity
  E. has antiarrhythmic activity.

14.151V An effective anthelmintic for dogs infested with:
  A. *Echinococcus granulosis* (hydatid tapeworm) is bunamidine
  B. *Toxocara canis* (dog roundworm) is piperazine
  C. *Ancylostoma caninum* (hookworm) is mebendazole
  D. *Dipylidium caninum* (flea tapeworm) is pyrantel
  E. *Dirofilaria immitis* (heartworm) is diethylcarbamazine.

14.152 Dichlorophen is:
  A. effective in nematode infestations
  B. effective in cestode infestations
  C. not effective in trematode infestations
  D. fungicidal
  E. poorly absorbed after oral administration.

14.153V Anticoccidial agents for use in chickens:
  A. must be used prophylactically
  B. are more effective at certain stages of parasite development
  C. can be coccidiostatic or coccidiocidal
  D. can be used effectively in doses that allow "controlled" infection
  E. are rarely administered as mixtures of two or three different agents.

14.154V Anticoccidial drugs useful in poultry farming include:
    A.   arecoline
    B.   sulphonamides
    C.   methyl benzoquate
    D.   amprolium hydrochloride
    E.   diaveridine.

14.155 Resistance of micro-organisms to penicillin can involve:
    A.   production of β-lactamase
    B.   loss of the cell wall under hypertonic conditions
    C.   exclusion of the drug because of alterations to the cell wall
    D.   transduction
    E.   production of an essential metabolite.

14.156 Penicillinase:
    A.   is a β-lactamase
    B.   hydrolyses benzylpenicillin to 6-aminopenicillanic acid
    C.   does not affect the β-lactam ring of cephaloridine
    D.   production is not responsible for the acquired resistance to methicillin exhibited by some staphylococci
    E.   inactivates carbenicillin.

14.157 Ampicillin:
    A.   is not inactivated by gastric acid
    B.   is subject to enterohepatic recycling
    C.   has a duration of action similar to that of benzylpenicillin
    D.   is as effective as benzylpenicillin against organisms sensitive to the latter
    E.   administered systemically is of little value in the treatment of mastitis.

14.158   A.   Benzylpenicillin is a useful antifungal agent.
    B.   Benzylpenicillin is the most potent of the penicillins *in vitro*.
    C.   Ampicillin is more acid-resistant then benzylpenicillin.
    D.   Both benzylpenicillin and ampicillin are sensitive to the enzyme penicillinase.
    E.   Benzylpenicillin has a short half life.

14.159 Aminoglycoside antibiotics may cause:
    A.   hypersensitivity
    B.   neurotoxicity
    C.   nephrotoxicity
    D.   neuromuscular blockade
    E.   agranulocytosis.

14.160 Aminoglycoside antibiotics:
    A.   are not absorbed from the gastrointestinal tract
    B.   are rapidly excreted in the urine
    C.   are bactericidal inhibitors of protein synthesis
    D.   are mainly active against gram-negative organisms
    E.   are subject to slowly-developing bacterial resistance.

14.161   A.   The spectrum of activity of tetracyclines overlaps that of penicillin and streptomycin and activity is often manifested against organisms resistant to both.

            B.   Tetracyclines bind reversibly to both ribosomes and m-RNA.

            C.   Resistance to tetracyclines is thought to depend on decreased uptake of antibiotic.

            D.   Tetracyclines are contraindicated in patients with renal dysfunction.

            E.   Development of photosensitivity limits the use of tetracyclines.

14.162 Chloramphenicol:
- A.   interferes with bacterial protein synthesis
- B.   may cause aplastic anaemia
- C.   has therapeutic and toxic effects which are not related
- D.   remains the drug of choice for the treatment of *Haemophilus influenzae* meningitis
- E.   remains the drug of choice for the treatment of *Salmonella* infections.

14.163 Flucytosine:
- A.   is actively transported into fungal cells
- B.   readily penetrates mammalian cells
- C.   is rapidly metabolised to 5-fluorouracil in fungal cells
- D.   is slowly metabolised to 5-fluorouracil in mammalian cells
- E.   is converted to an aberrant RNA.

14.164 Erythromycin:
- A.   blocks bacterial protein synthesis at the translocation step
- B.   can inhibit protein synthesis in mitochondria from mammalian cells
- C.   interferes with the binding of chloramphenicol to the ribosome
- D.   readily penetrates mammalian cell membranes
- E.   readily penetrates cell walls of gram-positive bacteria.

14.165 Unwanted effects of prolonged use of cancer chemotherapy drugs include:
- A.   dental caries
- B.   alopecia
- C.   intestinal ulcers
- D.   sterility
- E.   bone marrow depression.

14.166 Leukaemias may be treated by:
- A.   vincristine
- B.   methotrexate
- C.   chlorambucil
- D.   doxorubicin
- E.   erythromycin.

14.167 The effects of nitrogen mustards include:
- A.   anaemia
- B.   tissue damage at the site of injection
- C.   ulceration of the gastrointestinal tract
- D.   increased numbers of circulating platelets
- E.   increased susceptibility to infection.

14.168   Cis platinum produces the following side effects:
        A.   nausea and vomiting
        B.   pulmonary fibrosis
        C.   renal damage
        D.   ototoxicity
        E.   raised blood magnesium levels.

MCQ

14.169   Drug resistance in bacteria may involve:
        i.   production of antibiotic-degrading enzymes
        ii.   production of an essential metabolite
        iii.   morphological alterations which restrict the entry of the antibiotic into the cell
        iv.   altered metabolic pathways
        v.   transfer of extrachromosomal DNA.

14.170   In controlling the spread of multiply-resistant organisms, which of the following is/are of benefit?
        i.   isolation of known causes of infection
        ii.   hand washing
        iii.   antibiotic prescribing policies
        iv.   nasal swabs from all nursing, medical and ancillary staff
        v.   full barrier nursing of all intensive care patients.

14.171   Resistance of bacteria to an antibiotic may be overcome by the following stratagems:
        i.   long term, low dose therapy
        ii.   the use of antibiotic combinations
        iii.   intermittent therapy
        iv.   the use of an antibiotic of a different type
        v.   induction of enzymes in the host.

14.172   The major reasons for the concomitant use of two bactericidal antibiotics are:
        i.   drug synergism
        ii.   where the identity of the infecting organism(s) is unknown
        iii.   chance of bacterial resistance is reduced
        iv.   sensitivity reactions are less common
        v.   treatment time is lessened.

14.173   Penicillin acts by:
        i.   inhibition of DNA synthesis
        ii.   inhibition of cross linkage in the cell wall
        iii.   alteration of binding sites on sterols
        iv.   inhibition of a transpeptidase
        v.   altering the RNA template.

14.174   Acyclovir:
        i.   is active against viruses possessing thymidine kinase
        ii.   achieves effective tissue concentrations following intravenous administration
        iii.   is relatively non-toxic to mammalian cells which are not infected by viruses
        iv.   is active against measles virus
        v.   is poorly absorbed following oral administration.

14.175 Interferon:
    i.   is used in combination with idoxuridine to treat keratitis due to *Herpes simplex*
    ii.   has established its efficacy in the treatment of juvenile laryngeal papillomatosis
    iii.   inhibits multiplication of viruses.
    iv.   reduces the cytotoxicity of lymphocytes
    v.   is associated with few side effects because it is available in a highly purified form.

14.176 Simultaneous use of more than one drug is generally more effective than single agents for the treatment of cancer because:
    i.   cancer cells rapidly develop resistance to a single drug
    ii.   additional tumouricidal effects can be achieved
    iii.   very low doses of the drugs can be used
    iv.   within a single tumour, the cells vary in their susceptibility to different drugs
    v.   more frequent courses of treatment can be given.

14.177 Antimetabolites may exert their tumouricidal effects by:
    i.   inhibition of enzymes which mediate vital pathways for cell replication
    ii.   arresting cells in mitosis phase
    iii.   incorporation of antimetabolites as false bases in the synthesis of DNA and RNA
    iv.   intercalation of the drug between DNA chains
    v.   inhibition of nuclear receptor protein.

14.178 The side effects of doxorubicin include:
    i.   skin pigmentation
    ii.   dose-related cardiomyopathy
    iii.   Reynaud's phenomenon
    iv.   alopecia
    v.   peripheral neuropathy.

ASSERTION / REASON:

14.179 The combination of a sulphonamide with a folic acid synthesis inhibitor can confer a marked therapeutic advantage **BECAUSE** the combination of a sulphonamide with a folic acid synthesis inhibitor induces a sequential blockade of the metabolism of the invading organism.

14.180 Indiscriminate use of antibiotics in medicine and non-medical applications is a potential hazard to human health **BECAUSE** indiscriminate use of antibiotics increases the environmental load of antibiotic resistant bacteria, many of which are pathogenic to humans.

14.181 Multiply-resistant organisms are found principally in hospitals **BECAUSE** multiply-resistant organisms flourish in an antibiotic-rich environment.

14.182 When two bacteriostatic antibiotics are given together, synergism often occurs **BECAUSE** the attachment of two such antibiotics to ribosomes is mutually facilitated.

14.183 When a bactericidal antibiotic is administered after a bacteriostatic antibiotic, it is sometimes less effective than expected **BECAUSE** the decrease in bacterial metabolism which occurs after exposure to the bacteriostatic drug makes the organism less susceptible to the effect of the bactericidal drug.

14.184V If heartworm microfilariae are present in the circulation, administration of diethylcarbamazine to dogs may be hazardous **BECAUSE** the heartworm microfilariae killed by diethylcarbamazine may obstruct the pulmonary artery.

14.185 Severe infection in immunocompromised patients frequently fails to respond to antibiotics **BECAUSE** the natural defences of the body are at least as important as antibiotics in dealing with severe infection.

14.186 Primaquine prevents the occurrence of relapses of *Plasmodium falciparum* malaria **BECAUSE** primaquine has a lethal effect on dormant merozoites in the exo-erythrocyte stage of malaria.

14.187 In the treatment of acute attacks of malaria, chloroquine is preferred to pyrimethamine **BECAUSE** adverse effects are less likely to be produced by chloroquine than by pyrimethamine.

14.188 Emetine is the drug of choice for the treatment of amoebiasis **BECAUSE** emetine does not inhibit aldehyde dehydrogenase.

14.189 Mezlocillin must be administered by intravenous injection **BECAUSE** mezlocillin is not absorbed from the gastrointestinal tract.

14.190 Cephalosporins cannot be given to patients with a history of penicillin allergy **BECAUSE** cephalosporins have a more than 50% incidence of cross-reactivity in patients allergic to penicillin.

14.191 Potassium clavulanate potentiates the antibacterial activity of amoxycillin **BECAUSE** potassium clavulanate inhibits both excocellular and intracellular penicillinase.

14.192 Chloramphenicol should not be used to treat *Salmonella* infections **BECAUSE** bacterial resistance to chloramphenicol is readily transferred by means of extrachromosomal resistance factors.

14.193 The concurrent administration of aminoglycoside antibiotics and frusemide, decreases the incidence of ototoxicity **BECAUSE** both aminoglycoside antibiotics and frusemide are potentially ototoxic.

14.194 Griseofulvin is used in the treatment of some deep mycoses in man **BECAUSE** griseofulvin disrupts the incorporation of folic acid into fungal cell membranes.

14.195 Cytotoxic drugs may induce vomiting **BECAUSE** cytotoxic drugs directly stimulate the vomiting centre in the brain stem.

14.196 Vidarabine is used in the treatment of human viral encephalopathies **BECAUSE** vidarabine achieves concentrations in the cerebrospinal fluid which are greater than plasma levels.

ANSWERS

14.1	F	14.34	F	14.67	T	14.100	A	14.133	B	14.166	E
14.2	F	14.35	T	14.68	F	14.101	E	14.134	B	14.167	D
14.3	T	14.36	F	14.69	T	14.102	E	14.135	D	14.168	B
14.4	F	14.37	F	14.70	F	14.103	C	14.136	C	14.169	E
14.5	F	14.38	T	14.71	T	14.104	B	14.137	D	14.170	A
14.6	F	14.39	F	14.72	F	14.105	A	14.138	C	14.171	C
14.7	F	14.40	T	14.73	T	14.016	B	14.139	D	14.172	A
14.8	F	14.41	F	14.74	T	14.107	A	14.140	E	14.173	C
14.9	T	14.42	T	14.75	T	14.108	C	14.141	B	14.174	A
14.10	F	14.43	F	14.76	T	14.109	C	14.142	A	14.175	A
14.11	F	14.44	F	14.77	F	14.110	B	14.143	B	14.176	C
14.12	T	14.45	T	14.78	T	14.111	E	14.144	C	14.177	B
14.13	T	14.46	T	14.79	T	14.112	A	14.145	C	14.178	C
14.14	F	14.47	F	14.80	T	14.113	C	14.146	D	14.179	A
14.15	T	14.48	T	14.81	F	14.114	D	14.147	D	14.180	A
14.16	F	14.49	T	14.82	T	14.115	B	14.148	C	14.181	A
14.17	F	14.50	T	14.83	F	14.116	B	14.149	C	14.182	E
14.18	T	14.51	T	14.84	F	14.117	E	14.150	C	14.183	A
14.19	T	14.52	T	14.85	F	14.118	E	14.151	D	14.184	C
14.20	F	14.53	F	14.86	T	14.119	C	14.152	A	14.185	A
14.21	F	14.54	T	14.87	F	14.120	A	14.153	E	14.186	D
14.22	F	14.55	F	14.88	F	14.121	C	14.154	A	14.187	C
14.23	F	14.56	F	14.89	T	14.122	C	14.155	E	14.188	D
14.24	T	14.57	T	14.90	T	14.123	A	14.156	B	14.189	A
14.25	F	14.58	F	14.91	F	14.124	C	14.157	D	14.190	E
14.26	F	14.59	T	14.92	T	14.125	A	14.158	A	14.191	A
14.27	T	14.60	T	14.93	F	14.126	D	14.159	E	14.192	D
14.28	F	14.61	T	14.94	B	14.127	C	14.160	E	14.193	A
14.29	T	14.62	T	14.95	B	14.128	C	14.161	D	14.194	C
14.30	F	14.63	F	14.96	E	14.129	E	14.162	C	14.195	C
14.31	T	14.64	F	14.97	A	14.130	C	14.163	B	14.196	C
14.32	T	14.65	T	14.98	B	14.131	D	14.164	D		
14.33	F	14.66	T	14.99	D	14.132	B	14.165	A		

15 Drug Abuse

TRUE / FALSE

15.1   The development of tolerance to a central nervous system depressant begins with the first dose.

15.2   In Sydney metropolitan detoxification units where treatment is given for drug withdrawal, 90% of the patients are addicted to narcotic analgesics.

15.3   Nicotine is a drug of dependence.

15.4   Cocaine does not produce psychological dependency.

15.5   All sedative hypnotics possess the potential to produce physical dependence.

15.6   Physical dependence on diazepam does not occur.

15.7   The benzodiazepines do not produce psychological dependency.

15.8   Assuming a well-developed dependency, a life-threatening syndrome may occur on withdrawal of amylobarbitone.

15.9   Dependence on barbiturates is primarily due to alterations in liver metabolising function.

15.10 Ethanol, when taken in the fasting state, can induce hypoglycaemia.

15.11 The behavioural effects of ethanol are more marked when measured on the ascending phase of the blood ethanol curve than at the same point on the descending phase.

15.12 Conversion of acetaldehyde to acetate is the rate-limiting step in the metabolism of ethanol.

15.13 Metronidazole may block the metabolism of ethanol at the acetaldehyde stage.

15.14 Assuming a well-developed dependency, a syndrome of life-threatening severity may occur on the withdrawal of ethanol.

15.15 All manifestations of the withdrawal syndrome of an opioid can be terminated abruptly and dramatically by the administration of a suitable dose of that opioid.

15.16 Habitual use of morphine by pregnant women can result in the birth of physically dependent infants.

15.17   The most common cause of death from narcotic overdose is cerebral haemorrhage.

15.18   The time interval between successive doses of morphine is a very important determinant in the development of tolerance.

15.19   Tolerance to the narcotic drugs is due predominantly to changes in the rate of hepatic metabolism.

15.20   The degree of development of tolerance to the opioids is much greater than that to ethanol.

15.21   Physical dependence on heroin can develop in an individual who uses the drug only once a week.

15.22   Methadone is used in the treatment of morphine dependence.

15.23   The intensity of the narcotic withdrawal syndrome is independent of the degree of tolerance to the drug.

15.24   The peak severity of the withdrawal syndrome ('cold turkey') from morphine occurs about 2-3 days after withdrawal of the drug.

15.25   The withdrawal syndrome from methadone is of more sudden onset than that which occurs from an equivalent dependency to heroin.

15.26   Assuming a similar degree of dependence, the severity of the withdrawal syndrome with heroin is greater than that with methadone.

15.27   Clonidine has been found to be clinically useful in alleviating the intensity of the narcotic withdrawal syndrome.

15.28   The severity of the narcotic withdrawal syndrome is directly related to the magnitude of the doses which were taken.

15.29   The naloxone pupil test is a means for detecting narcotic dependence in patients.

15.30   Cannabis preparations are effective in the treatment of glaucoma.

15.31   Cannabidiol does not possess mood-altering properties.

15.32   Violent behaviour is more likely to be a consequence of the effects of ethanol than of cannabis.

15.33   Cannabis causes marked short-term memory failure.

15.34   Δ-9-Tetrahydrocannabinol may precipitate fitting in epileptic patients.

15.35   Tolerance does not occur to cannabis preparations.

15.36   Heavy users of cannabis can become psychologically dependent on the drug.

15.37   Assuming a well-developed dependency, a life-threatening syndrome may occur on withdrawal of cannabis.

15.38   A cannabis withdrawal syndrome has been demonstrated to occur in man.

15.39   Many hallucinogens are structurally related to 5-hydroxytryptamine.

15.40   Mescaline exhibits cross-tolerance to lysergic acid diethylamide (LSD).

15.41   Cross-tolerance exists between the hallucinogenic properties of lysergic acid diethylamide (LSD) and Δ-9-tetrahydrocannabinol.

15.42   The hallucinogenic dose of lysergic acid diethylamide (LSD) is dangerously close to that which produces respiratory depression.

CORRECT OPTION

15.43   Which of the following may not be associated with a withdrawal syndrome?
    A.   ethanol
    B.   caffeine
    C.   mescaline
    D.   diazepam
    E.   nicotine.

15.44   Ethanol can most markedly potentiate the toxic effects of:
    A.   antiarrhythmic drugs
    B.   antimalarials
    C.   barbiturates
    D.   disodium cromoglycate
    E.   heavy metals.

15.45   The legally prescribed blood ethanol limit for drivers of motor vehicles in New South Wales is:
    A.   0.8 gm/100 ml
    B.   0.5 gm/100 ml
    C.   0.1 gm/100 ml
    D.   0.08 gm/100 ml
    E.   0.05 gm/100 ml.

15.46   The maximum number of 285 ml glasses (N.S.W. middies) of normal strength beer which can be consumed in one hour by a normal healthy 70 kg adult in the fasted state and still remain below the N.S.W. legal blood ethanol limit for drivers is:
    A.   1
    B.   3
    C.   5
    D.   7
    E.   9.

15.47   The legally prescribed blood ethanol limit for drivers is based upon evidence derived from:
    A.   laboratory studies based on human performance
    B.   studies using a driving simulator
    C.   epidemiological studies of road crashes
    D.   an assessment of the socially acceptable level of drunkenness.

15.48   The average rate of disappearance of ethanol from the blood once drinking
        has stopped is:
        A.   0.015 mg ethanol/100 ml blood/hour
        B.   0.15 mg ethanol/100 ml blood/hour
        C.   0.015 g ethanol/100 ml blood/hour
        D.   0.15 g ethanol/100 ml blood/hour.

15.49   The elimination rate of ethanol can be increased by:
        A.   exercise
        B.   drinking coffee
        C.   drinking water
        D.   carbonation of the ethanolic beverage
        E.   none of the above.

15.50   The principal psychoactive component of cannabis is:
        A.   cannabinol
        B.   cannabidiol
        C.   nabilone
        D.   Δ-9-tetrahydrocannabinol.

15.51   The interaction between cannabis and ethanol as it affects human
        psychomotor performance is:
        A.   additive
        B.   potentiative
        C.   antagonistic
        D.   metabolic
        E.   none of the above.

15.52   The major route of elimination of ethanol in humans is:
        A.   oxidation in the blood
        B.   excretion *via* the kidneys and lungs
        C.   oxidation in the liver
        D.   excretion *via* the bile duct.

15.53   Which of the following statements is correct?
        A.   Metronidazole accelerates the metabolism of ethanol.
        B.   The central nervous system depressant effects of ethanol and
             diazepam are synergistic.
        C.   Caffeine antagonises all the inebriant effects of ethanol.
        D.   All antihistamines increase the central nervous system
             depressant effects of ethanol.
        E.   Δ-9-Tetrahydrocannabinol has no interactive effect with ethanol.

MCQ

15.54   Abuse of which of the following drugs may cause marked physical
        dependence?
        i.   diazepam
        ii.   pentobarbitone
        iii.   morphine
        iv.   amphetamine
        v.   cannabis.

15.55   Which of the following drugs may interact with alcohol to impair driving
         skills?
        i.   antihistamines
        ii.   antidepressants
        iii.   cannabis
        iv.   sedatives
        v.   tranquillisers.

ASSERTION / REASON

15.56   LSD-induced hallucinatory episodes closely imitate those experienced in
         true schizophrenia **BECAUSE** LSD-induced hallucinations are
         predominantly auditory.

15.57   Aspirin is a causative factor in many road crashes **BECAUSE** aspirin is a
         drug which is commonly consumed by a large proportion of drivers.

15.58   The "legal" limit for blood ethanol in drivers in New South Wales has been
         set at 0.05 gm/100 ml **BECAUSE** 25% of drivers with a blood ethanol level of
         0.05 gm/100 ml are involved in traffic crashes.

ANSWERS

15.1	T	15.13	T	15.25	F	15.37	F	15.49	E
15.2	F	15.14	T	15.26	T	15.38	T	15.50	D
15.3	T	15.15	T	15.27	T	15.39	T	15.51	A
15.4	F	15.16	T	15.28	T	15.40	T	15.52	C
15.5	T	15.17	F	15.29	T	15.41	F	15.53	B
15.6	F	15.18	T	15.30	T	15.42	F	15.54	A
15.7	F	15.19	F	15.31	T	15.43	C	15.55	E
15.8	T	15.20	T	15.32	T	15.44	C	15.56	E
15.9	F	15.21	F	15.33	T	15.45	E	15.57	D
15.10	T	15.22	T	15.34	T	15.46	B	15.58	C
15.11	T	15.23	F	15.35	F	15.47	C		
15.12	F	15.24	T	15.36	T	15.48	C		

16 Toxicology

TRUE / FALSE

16.1   Toxic properties of drugs may be exhibited by functional, biochemical or structural changes .

16.2   The site of accumulation of a chemical in the body is not necessarily the target organ of the toxic response.

16.3   An antidote may displace a toxic substance from susceptible binding sites.

16.4   An antidote to a drug overdose must act as a competitive antagonist to the drug.

16.5   The most rational antidotal therapy for envenomation by noxious animals is administration of an appropriate antivenom.

16.6   The liver has a large capacity to regenerate after chemically-induced damage.

16.7   Clearly identifiable threshold levels, below which toxic effects do not occur, have been established for most environmental toxins.

16.8   Ascending paralysis following administration of a neurotoxin is unequivocal evidence for a central site of action.

16.9V   Hepatotoxins which result in bile duct obstruction may initiate secondary photosensitisation.

16.10   All snake venom phospholipases are presynaptic neurotoxins.

16.11   The penetration of mercury into living tissue depends on its oxidation state.

16.12   Silicosis is associated with cytotoxicity to alveolar macrophages.

16.13   Alkyl mercury compounds can be synthesised by aquatic micro-organisms and incorporated into the food chain.

16.14   D-Penicillamine produces less inherent toxic responses than dimercaprol when used as an antidote to poisoning by mercurial compounds.

16.15   Thalidomide was withdrawn from use because of its mutagenic action in pregnant women.

16.16   Kerosene poisoning can effectively be treated by emesis.

16.17 Ingestion of turpentine requires immediate induction of emesis.

16.18 Selective injury to the retinal cells by excess methanol ingestion is thought to be caused by the toxic metabolite, formic acid.

16.19 Emetic agents are contraindicated when children have ingested corrosive acids or alkalis.

16.20 When hydrochloric acid is swallowed, the recommended treatment is two teaspoons of sodium bicarbonate in a glass of water.

16.21 Cobalt edetate is a potentially useful chelating agent for the treatment of cyanide intoxication.

16.22 Dimercaprol is an effective antidote for selenium poisoning.

16.23 Dimercaprol is an antidote to poisoning by organic arsenicals and arsenic salts.

16.24 The delayed onset of symptoms distinguishes arsenic from other metallic poisons.

16.25 Benzene inhibits blood cell formation in the bone marrow.

16.26 DDT, like other chlorinated hydrocarbons, is well absorbed from the skin.

16.27 Pyrethrins and DDT modify sodium channels on nerve fibres.

16.28 When organophosphorus insecticides interact with acetylcholinesterase, "aging" of the phosphorylated enzyme gradually makes the phosphorylation step irreversible.

16.29 Salicylate overdose in children under six years causes a mild acid-base disturbance which is of little medical consequence.

16.30 After the ingestion of toxic doses of aspirin, there is a decrease in the peripheral utilisation of oxygen and a consequent decrease in carbon dioxide production in peripheral tissues.

16.31 Hepatotoxicity may occur after ingestion of 20 mg of paracetamol.

16.32 The hepatotoxicity of paracetamol can be reduced with N-acetylcysteine.

16.33 Fatal liver damage due to paracetamol overdosage may be prevented by the administration of diethylmaleate within 24 hours of ingestion of the paracetamol.

16.34 Tetraethyl lead emitted from automobile exhaust is the major contributing factor to the blood lead level of an average adult urban dweller.

16.35 In the bloodstream, up to 90% of absorbed lead is bound to plasma proteins.

16.36 Excessive blood lead levels can be effectively treated with penicillin therapy.

16.37 Lead is found in higher concentrations in white blood cells than in red blood cells.

16.38 Lead poisoning leads to elevated levels of copper, iron and zinc in the brain.

16.39V Chronic lead poisoning in the dog may lead to multiple convulsive seizures.

16.40V The haemolytic crisis of copper poisoning in sheep is associated with loss of glutathione from the erythrocyte membrane.

16.41V Inorganic arsenites will be absorbed from the skin only if it is abraded.

16.42 Chronic administration of arsenic leads to accumulation in tissue keratin.

16.43 Toxic doses of arsenic salts do not affect gastrointestinal function.

16.44V Ducks may be poisoned after eating molluscoid baits containing metaldehyde.

16.45V Metaldehyde-induced convulsions in domestic animals are commonly controlled by diazepam and supportive treatment.

16.46 Warfarin poisoning in domestic animals can be effectively treated with vitamin K preparations.

16.47V The cyanogenic principle in bracken fern frequently causes poisoning in horses and cattle.

16.48V The concentration of nitrates and cyanogenic glycosides in plants may increase following application of the herbicide 2,4-D.

16.49V Cyanogenic glycosides rarely occur in Australian native plants.

16.50V The pyrrolizidine alkaloids found in *Heliotropium europaeum* can trigger a haemolytic crisis similar to that evoked by chronic phytogenous copper ingestion.

16.51V Lupinosis in sheep is associated with the alkaloids lupinine and sparteine.

16.52V Acute poisoning of sheep by lupins is almost invariably fatal.

16.53V St. George disease in cattle following chronic ingestion of *Pimelia* species is characterised by cardiac failure and increased pulmonary vascular resistance.

16.54V Poisoning of horses by Crofton weed (*Eupatorium adenophorum*) occurs only in the Lismore area of New South Wales.

16.55V In the horse, the target organ for the toxic principles of *Eupatorium adenophorum* (Crofton weed) is the lung.

16.56V Although its effects are usually seen in horses, Crofton weed (*Eupatorium adenophorum*) occasionally affects cattle.

16.57V Facial eczema in sheep is produced when perennial rye grass infected with *Phomopsis leptostromoformis* is consumed.

16.58V Facial eczema in sheep is a photosensitivity reaction caused by deposition of sporidesmin in exposed skin.

16.59V Hypericin causes hypersensitivity reactions in animals secondary to its hepatotoxic action.

16.60V Chronic *Phalaris* poisoning generally involves irreversible lesions in the central nervous system.

16.61V Sheep are more susceptible to *Senecio* poisoning than horses.

16.62V Aspirin is more toxic to the dog than to the cat.

CORRECT OPTION

16.63 The threshold limit value (TLV) defines a safe:
    A.   daily intake of food additives
    B.   ambient air concentrations of chemicals found in the workplace
    C.   water content of heavy metals
    D.   concentration of excipient in therapeutic drugs.

16.64 Toxic effects of compounds on the foetus are dependent upon:
    A.   the inherent toxicity of the compound
    B.   renal elimination of the compound
    C.   glucuronyl transferase activity
    D.   the developmental stage of the foetus
    E.   all of the above.

16.65 Which of the following is not a common component of air pollution?
    A.   sulphur oxides
    B.   carbon dioxide
    C.   hydrocarbons
    D.   nitrogen oxides.

16.66 The venom of the funnel-web spider is:
    A.   toxic to all species
    B.   not toxic to man
    C.   toxic to primates only
    D.   none of the above.

16.67 An important difference between short and long chain α-toxins in snake venom is:
    A.   short chain toxins block acetylcholine release while long chain toxins block acetylcholine receptors
    B.   short chain toxins block nicotinic receptors while long chain toxins block muscarinic receptors
    C.   short chain toxins bind to human acetylcholine receptors while long chain toxins do not
    D.   long chain toxins bind to human acetylcholine receptors while short chain toxins do not
    E.   short chain toxins are all phospholipases while long chain toxins are not.

16.68   Haemolysis by snake venoms:
    A.   is caused by α-toxins
    B.   is the result of direct degradation of membrane lipids only
    C.   is the result of direct degradation of membrane lipids and the effects of lysolecithin
    D.   is the result of the effects of lysolecithin only.

16.69   Death from snake bite in Australia results primarily from:
    A.   respiratory failure
    B.   thromboses
    C.   heart block
    D.   tissue necrosis
    E.   action on the central nervous system.

16.70   An important factor contributing to the effectiveness of chelation therapy in metal poisoning is that:
    A.   chelated metals are readily metabolised in the liver
    B.   chelated metals are water soluble
    C.   chelated metals are lipid soluble
    D.   chelating agents facilitate the binding of metals to plasma proteins.

16.71   Which of the following metal poisonings should not be treated by chelation therapy?
    A.   arsenic
    B.   lead
    C.   cadmium
    D.   mercury
    E.   copper.

16.72   Which of the following is not characteristic of lead poisoning?
    A.   pallor
    B.   colic
    C.   "milk and roses" complexion
    D.   constipation
    E.   anaemia.

16.73   In cases of poisoning by iron salts, the preferred antidote is:
    A.   dimercaprol
    B.   calcium sodium edetate
    C.   D-penicillamine
    D.   desferrioxamine
    E.   pralidoxime.

16.74   Minimata disease describes:
    A.   the central and peripheral nervous system lesions associated with methylmercury poisoning
    B.   a zinc deficiency disease found only in Japan
    C.   a bone disease resulting from exposure to mercury
    D.   a muscle wasting disease which follows snake bite.

16.75   The toxicity of heavy metals depends on:
    A.   nutritional status
    B.   concurrent intake of other metals
    C.   concurrent consumption of drugs
    D.   all of the above.

16.76 Which of the following substances is not stored in the matrix of the bone?
    A. strontium
    B. arsenic
    C. fluoride
    D. lead.

16.77 Which of the following metals causes poisoning with symptoms resembling Guillain-Barre syndrome?
    A. copper
    B. lead
    C. iron
    D. arsenic
    E. mercury.

16.78 Which of the following side effects is not associated with an acute overdose of protriptyline?
    A. hyperpyrexia
    B. hypotension
    C. hypertension
    D. convulsions
    E. salivation.

16.79 Hazards associated with excess aspirin ingestion in children include:
    A. hypothermia
    B. respiratory alkalosis
    C. metabolic alkalosis
    D. oedema
    E. all of the above.

16.80 The cause of death in salicylate poisoning is:
    A. hyperventilation
    B. tinnitus
    C. respiratory depression
    D. liver damage.

16.81 Which of the following drug groups is most commonly encountered in human poisoning fatalities?
    A. anticonvulsants
    B. analgesics
    C. sedative hypnotics
    D. antidepressants
    E. antipsychotics.

16.82 Death is most frequently associated with illicit use of:
    A. LSD
    B. amphetamine
    C. heroin
    D. cannabis
    E. methadone.

16.83 The tablets inducing the least severe toxic reaction in children under five years of age are:
    A. antidepressants
    B. ferrous sulphate
    C. oral contraceptives
    D. aspirin.

16.84   Ethanol causes significant potentiation of the toxic effects of:
    A.   carbon monoxide
    B.   barbiturates
    C.   heavy metals
    D.   antimalarial drugs
    E.   antiarrhythmic drugs.

16.85   Reversal of severe respiratory depression can be achieved with an intravenous injection of naloxone following poisoning with:
    A.   aminopyrine
    B.   methadone
    C.   phenylbutazone
    D.   indomethacin
    E.   lignocaine.

16.86   An increase in the incidence of cancer, particularly in smokers, is associated with chronic exposure to:
    A.   talc
    B.   asbestos
    C.   silica
    D.   cobalt.

16.87   The cause of death in acute paracetamol overdose is:
    A.   acute liver failure
    B.   methaemoglobinaemia
    C.   haemolysis
    D.   convulsions
    E.   failure of blood coagulation mechanisms.

16.88   A promising method of prevention of hepatotoxicity after paracetamol overdosage is:
    A.   phototherapy
    B.   phenobarbitone administration
    C.   albumin infusion
    D.   N-acetylcysteine administration
    E.   none of the above.

16.89   DDT:
    A.   is absorbed through skin
    B.   inactivates cholinesterase in insects
    C.   induces metabolism and detoxification of barbiturates
    D.   has a short half-life in mammals
    E.   induces carcinogenic responses after chronic exposure.

16.90   Botulinum poisoning:
    A.   can be reversed by anticholinesterases
    B.   only affects the elderly
    C.   is reversed by growth of new motor terminals
    D.   is characterised by massive haemolysis.

16.91   Piperonyl butoxide is added to insecticides to:
         A.   prevent photochemical breakdown of pyrethrins
         B.   potentiate the actions of pyrethrins by inhibiting mixed function oxidase activity
         C.   potentiate the actions of organophosphates by inhibiting mixed function oxidase activity
         D.   potentiate the actions of pyrethrins by increasing the lipid solubility of the insecticide
         E.   decrease the mammalian toxicity of the organophosphates by inhibiting the metabolic activation process.

16.92   Which route of exposure to carbon tetrachloride allows the most rapid absorption?
         A.   oral ingestion
         B.   inhalation
         C.   subcutaneous injection
         D.   topical application to the skin.

16.93 - 16.96

16.93   antimalarials

16.94   C-17 substituted testosterone derivatives

16.95   halothane

16.96   chlorpromazine

For each of the drugs listed above, indicate whether its toxicity depends on:

         A.   decreased intracanalicular transport of bilirubin
         B.   direct hepatocellular damage
         C.   increased red blood cell destruction and consequent increase in bilirubin load for the liver
         D.   decreased acetylation due to genetic determinants.

16.97 - 16.100

16.97   sodium edetate

16.98   D-penicillamine

16.99   dimercaprol

16.100   desferrioxamine

For each of the compounds listed above, indicate whether it is most appropriate for the treatment of poisoning by:

         A.   iron
         B.   calcium
         C.   arsenic
         D.   copper.

16.101   The recommended upper limit of lead in the blood of children is:
      A. 2 µg/100 ml
      B. 10 µg/100 ml
      C. 30 µg/100 ml
      D. 100 µg/100 ml.

16.102V Plants associated with nitrate poisoning in grazing animals include:
      A. white heliotrope
      B. rhubarb leaves
      C. oats
      D. bracken fern
      E. sorghum.

16.103V The chief effects of bracken poisoning in horses may be attributed to:
      A. an aplastic anaemia factor
      B. cyanogenic glycosides
      C. thiaminase
      D. a carcinogenic factor.

16.104V Bracken fern contains many toxic components including:
      A. a photosensitiser
      B. an aplastic anaemia factor
      C. a goitrogen
      D. thiamine analogues.

16.105V The greatest phytoestrogen hazard to sheep is in pasture plants containing predominantly:
      A. coumestrol
      B. formononetin
      C. genistein
      D. biochanin A.

INCORRECT OPTION

16.106V Target organs for the toxic effects of oxalate ions include:
      A. brain
      B. liver
      C. kidney
      D. erythrocytes.

16.107   Photosensitivity reactions may occur in patients using the following drugs and then exposing themselves to bright sunlight:
      A. tricyclic antidepressants
      B. phenothiazine tranquillisers
      C. methylated p-amino benzoic acid derivatives
      D. thiazide diuretics.

16.108   Delayed toxicity is exhibited by:
      A. benzene
      B. chloramphenicol
      C. ferrous sulphate
      D. paraquat.

16.109   Specific antidotes are available for the treatment of poisoning by:
    A. selenium
    B. arsenic
    C. lead
    D. mercury.

16.110   Toxic effects of paracetamol include:
    A. respiratory depression
    B. methaemoglobinaemia
    C. tinnitus
    D. hepatic coma
    E. cardiovascular collapse.

16.111   The symptoms of lead poisoning:
    A. only develop after long-term ingestion
    B. include effects on haem enzymes
    C. are generally difficult to identify in patients with blood lead levels of 40 µg/100 ml
    D. include peripheral neuropathies
    E. can be usefully treated with chelating agents.

16.112   Tetraethyl lead:
    A. can be absorbed directly through the skin
    B. is not poisonous because it is an organo-lead derivative
    C. is concentrated in the kidney and liver
    D. is slowly converted to inorganic lead in the body
    E. crosses the blood-brain barrier more easily than inorganic lead.

16.113   The following factors have an important bearing on the toxicity of lead:
    A. age
    B. species
    C. sex
    D. pregnancy.

16.114   Concerning lead:
    A. Blood lead levels give an indication of recent exposure to lead.
    B. Bone can contain 90% of the total body burden of lead.
    C. In the general population, the major proportion of an individual's blood lead can be directly attributed to inhaled lead from automobile exhausts.
    D. Atmospheric lead levels normally decrease rapidly with distance from major traffic routes.
    E. Lead can inhibit enzymes concerned with haem synthesis.

16.115V Pyrrolizidine alkaloids have been responsible for:
    A. photosensitivity
    B. disrupted copper storage
    C. haemolytic jaundice
    D. depression of protein synthesis.

16.116V Pyrrolizidine alkaloids in heliotrope may cause the following effects in sheep:
    A. sudden death through acute ammonia intoxication
    B. haemolytic crisis of chronic copper poisoning
    C. emaciation due to hepatic failure
    D. primary photosensitisation.

16.117V The toxic effects of pyrrolizidine alkaloids:
- A. are most commonly observed in sheep and horses
- B. may cause photosensitivity reactions
- C. may resemble low molybdenum ingestion in sheep
- D. stimulate parenchymal mitosis in the liver.

16.118V Mycotoxins are fungal metabolites and include:
- A. zearalenone
- B. sparteine
- C. aflatoxin B1
- D. sporidesmin
- E. toxins from *Phomopsis leptostromoformis*.

16.119V Acute *Phalaris* toxicity in sheep is associated with:
- A. gramine
- B. 5-methoxydimethyltryptamine
- C. ergotamine
- D. bufotenine.

16.120V The toxic effects of alkaloids from *Solanum* species include:
- A. mucosal irritation in the intestine
- B. haemolysis
- C. haemoglobinuria
- D. central nervous stimulation
- E. tachycardia followed by bradycardia.

16.121 Sanguinarine, an isoquinoline alkaloid which occurs in seeds of *Argemone mexicana* (Mexican poppy), has the following effects in chickens:
- A. increased egg production
- B. haemorrhagic enteritis
- C. inhibition of brain pyruvate oxidation
- D. cyanosis of the comb.

16.122V Solanaceous alkaloids include:
- A. nicotine
- B. retrorscine
- C. hyoscyamine
- D. solanidine.

16.123V Symptoms associated with selenium poisoning in horses include:
- A. diarrhoea
- B. malaise
- C. depilation of mane and tail
- D. hoof deformities.

MCQ

16.124 Australian snake venoms contain a multitude of components which typically may include:
- i. anticoagulants
- ii. convulsant proteins and polypeptides
- iii. phospholipase A
- iv. monoamine oxidase inhibitors.

16.125 Which of the following statements concerning paracetamol toxicity is/are correct?
    i.   The formation of the active metabolite requires previously induced microsomal enzymes.
    ii.   Plasma concentrations of the drug measured shortly after ingestion help predict the risk of toxicity.
    iii. Pre-existing liver disease (e.g. hepatitis) increases the risk of toxicity.
    iv. Sulphydryl-containing compounds (cysteamine, N-acetylcysteine) are useful in the management of paracetamol toxicity.

16.126 Acetylcholinesterase inhibitory effects are exhibited by:
    i.   chlorinated hydrocarbon pesticides eg. DDT
    ii.   quaternary ammonium herbicides eg. paraquat
    iii. phenoxyacid herbicides eg. 2,4-D
    iv. organophosphate insecticides eg. parathion
    v.   alkaloids eg. strychnine.

16.127 Symptoms of poisoning by organophosphorus insecticides include:
    i.   pupil constriction
    ii.   bradycardia
    iii. vomiting and diarrhoea
    iv. salivation
    v.   bronchoconstriction.

16.128V Chronic toxic effects of alkyl derivatives of mercury in cats include:
    i.   loss of the righting reflex
    ii.   posterior weakness
    iii. hypersalivation
    iv. tonic-clonic convulsions
    v.   vocal indications of distress.

ASSERTION/REASON

16.129 Children are more susceptible to lead poisoning than adults **BECAUSE** most neurones in the human brain are formed after birth.

16.130 Deltamethrin is a more useful insecticide than the natural pyrethrins **BECAUSE** deltamethrin has improved stability to light and to oxidation compared to the natural pyrethrins.

16.131 Paracetamol, in conventional therapeutic doses, should not be given to patients with liver disease **BECAUSE** paracetamol in large doses causes hepatic necrosis.

ANSWERS

16.1	T	16.23	T	16.45	T	16.67	D	16.89	C	16.111	A
16.2	T	16.24	F	16.46	T	16.68	C	16.90	C	16.112	E
16.3	T	16.25	T	16.47	F	16.69	A	16.91	B	16.113	C
16.4	F	16.26	F	16.48	T	16.70	B	16.92	B	16.114	C
16.5	T	16.27	T	16.49	F	16.71	A	16.93	C	16.115	D
16.6	T	16.28	T	16.50	T	16.72	C	16.94	A	16.116	D
16.7	F	16.29	F	16.51	F	16.73	D	16.95	B	16.117	D
16.8	F	16.30	F	16.52	F	16.74	A	16.96	A	16.118	B
16.9	T	16.31	T	16.53	T	16.75	D	16.97	B	16.119	C
16.10	F	16.32	T	16.54	F	16.76	B	16.98	D	16.120	D
16.11	T	16.33	F	16.55	T	16.77	B	16.99	C	16.121	A
16.12	T	16.34	F	16.56	F	16.78	A	16.100	A	16.122	B
16.13	T	16.35	F	16.57	F	16.79	B	16.101	C	16.123	A
16.14	T	16.36	F	16.58	F	16.80	C	16.102	C	16.124	B
16.15	F	16.37	F	16.59	F	16.81	C	16.103	C	16.125	C
16.16	F	16.38	F	16.60	T	16.82	C	16.104	B	16.126	D
16.17	F	16.39	T	16.61	F	16.83	C	16.105	B	16.127	E
16.18	F	16.40	T	16.62	F	16.84	B	16.106	B	16.128	E
16.19	T	16.41	F	16.63	B	16.85	B	16.107	C	16.129	C
16.20	F	16.42	T	16.64	E	16.86	B	16.108	C	16.130	A
16.21	T	16.43	F	16.65	B	16.87	A	16.109	A	16.131	D
16.22	F	16.44	T	16.66	C	16.88	D	16.110	C		

17 Drug Development and Registration

TRUE / FALSE

17.1 While it is satisfactory to allow a few falsely positive or active compounds to enter final drug screening, it is not satisfactory to eliminate active compounds.

17.2 The ambient temperature of a laboratory is of no significance in the conduct of an experiment using phenothiazines in mice.

17.3 Suppression of pentylenetetrazole-induced seizures in mice is a useful model for assessing drugs with potential activity in petit mal epilepsy in humans.

17.4 Isolated guinea-pig atria are useful and specific preparations to test for β_1-adrenoceptor agonist activity.

17.5 A well-designed clinical trial always includes an inactive placebo.

17.6 In a double-blind clinical trial neither the observer nor the subject knows which medication has been administered.

17.7 A properly controlled clinical trial will always reveal potential side effects.

17.8 Section B2 of a general marketing application for a new drug contains the detailed reports of animal studies.

17.9 The period of chronic toxicity testing for a new drug depends on the intended use of that drug.

17.10 In Australia, all drugs which are introduced into medicine must undergo local clinical trials.

17.11 There is a definite relationship between the incidence and/or severity of side effects tolerable in a new drug and the severity of the condition it is supposed to ameliorate.

17.12 In Australia, once a new drug is approved for marketing, the pharmaceutical company's obligation for post-marketing reporting to the Department of Health is limited to notification of suspected adverse drug reaction reports for three years.

17.13 Before an adverse reaction is reported to the Australian Drug Evaluation Committee, the physician must establish a definite link between drug and effect.

CORRECT OPTION

17.14 The toad rectus abdominis preparation is suitable for the investigation of drugs which act on:
    A.   β-adrenoceptors
    B.   α- and β-adrenoceptors
    C.   muscarinic receptors
    D.   nicotinic receptors
    E.   histamine receptors.

17.15 In the screening of drugs for topical local anaesthetic action, the most appropriate screening method is:
    A.   the mouse tail flick method
    B.   the guinea pig wheal method
    C.   the rabbit eye method
    D.   the rectal probe method
    E.   the hot plate method.

17.16 The isolated guinea-pig ileum preparation is useful for detecting compounds with:
    A.   antimuscarinic activity
    B.   α-adrenoceptor antagonist activity
    C.   β-adrenoceptor antagonist activity
    D.   reserpine-like activity
    E.   none of the above.

17.17 Sooper-Dooper laboratories have isolated a hitherto unknown substance from fruit-bat wings. Because it was effective in suppressing antigen-induced bronchoconstriction in sensitised guinea-pigs, the chief pharmacologist concluded that it may have properties similar to:
    A.   mepyramine
    B.   cimetidine
    C.   disodium cromoglycate
    D.   dexamethasone
    E.   aminophylline.

17.18 A distinguishing feature of the Phase III clinical trial programme is that:
    A.   subjects are generally healthy volunteers
    B.   establishment of efficacy relative to placebo is the objective of most studies
    C.   approximately 200 subjects are involved
    D.   general practitioners are always involved
    E.   long term safety is of major concern.

17.19 The cross-over clinical trial design:
    A.   is restricted in its use to acute disease which is self-limiting in its course
    B.   is unsuitable for a double-blind, placebo controlled study
    C.   may not be used when making a double-blind comparison of two drugs using the double dummy technique
    D.   requires larger patient numbers than the two parallel group design
    E.   is most valid in a chronic condition without marked fluctuations in intensity.

17.20   The Ames test tests a drug for:
      A.   pulmonary toxicity
      B.   carcinogenicity of the parent drug
      C.   hepatotoxicity
      D.   mutagenicity of hepatic metabolites
      E.   nephrotoxicity.

17.21   The only practical test at present for detecting point mutation in a mammalian test system is:
      A.   the Ames test
      B.   dominant lethal assays
      C.   *in vivo* cytogenic assays
      D.   host-mediated assays.

17.22   Which test is most likely to provide an accurate prediction of the potential carcinogenicity of a chemical?
      A.   90 day sub-acute study in the beagle dog
      B.   3-generation rat reproduction study
      C.   mutagenicity tests using *Salmonella* strains
      D.   2 year rat chronic feeding study.

ANSWERS

17.1	T	17.6	T	17.11	T	17.16	A	17.21	A
17.2	F	17.7	F	17.12	F	17.17	C	17.22	D
17.3	T	17.8	T	17.13	F	17.18	E		
17.4	T	17.9	T	17.14	D	17.19	E		
17.5	F	17.10	F	17.15	C	17.20	B		

18 Theory of Practical Experiments

TRUE / FALSE

18.1 Biological variation is the only source of experimental error in any bioassay.

18.2 The standard error is an estimate of the degree of variability of the mean of a sample.

18.3 In a statistical comparison of sample means, the level of significance is the probability value above which the null hypothesis is accepted.

18.4 Linear regression is a statistical procedure used to find the straight line that best fits a set of data points.

18.5 The chi-square test is used for quantal data.

18.6 The Student t-test always assumes observations are drawn from a normally distributed population.

18.7 Two samples are compared by Student's t-test to determine whether they are significantly different at the 0.05 level. If P=0.03, the two samples are considered to be significantly different.

18.8 A t-value of 2.0 is calculated from the comparison of the mean weights of two groups of mice. (From the tables, the critical value of t corresponding to P = 0.05 is 2.1.) This indicates that the mean weights are significantly different.

18.9 The Mann-Whitney U-test is a parametric test of significance of the difference between two means.

18.10 A Mann-Whitney U-test should only be used when the data are normally distributed.

18.11 Probit analysis is a statistical technique for evaluating quantal log dose-response data.

18.12 Probit analysis transforms the sigmoid log dose-response curve into a straight line.

18.13 The slope of a log dose-probit line for a given drug is independent of the biological variation in sensitivity to that drug.

18.14 As the magnitude of the 95% confidence limits increases, the reliability of the bioassay is increased.

18.15   The pA_2 value is a measure of the potency of an agonist drug.

18.16   The maximal contraction of a guinea-pig ileum elicited by acetylcholine is larger than that elicited by choline.

18.17   In high doses, mepyramine can have atropine-like effects.

18.18   Nicotine is a more potent agonist than acetylcholine in the isolated guinea-pig ileum.

18.19   Nicotine, in high doses, can "block" nicotinic receptors in the isolated guinea-pig ileum preparation.

18.20   In isolated guinea-pig atria, carbachol increases both the rate and force of contraction.

18.21   Quinidine increases the maximum frequency at which isolated atria can be electrically paced.

18.22   Ouabain and related glycosides increase the rate of atrial beating by inhibition of the Na^+, K^+-ATPase pump.

18.23   Tricyclic antidepressants potentiate the effects of isoprenaline in the isolated rabbit jejunum preparation.

18.24   Phentolamine reduces the effect of noradrenaline on the rabbit jejunum.

18.25   Guanethidine, in the presence of amitriptyline, decreases the spontaneous contractions of the rabbit jejunum.

18.26   Pretreatment of the rabbit jejunum with guanethidine reduces the effect of isoprenaline.

18.27   Salbutamol competitively inhibits acetylcholine-induced contractions of the isolated rat uterus.

18.28   In the isolated rat uterus preparation, the onset of action of oxytocin is more rapid than that of acetylcholine.

18.29   Ergometrine produces a rhythmic contractile-relaxant response in the oestrogen-primed rat uterus preparation.

18.30   The neuromuscular blocking action of suxamethonium is reversed by neostigmine.

18.31   If acetylcholine is incubated in a mixture of neostigmine in serum, a dose of the incubate will produce a contraction on the toad rectus abdominis preparation.

18.32   Pretreating animals with neostigmine increases the ED_{50} of (+)-tubocurarine.

18.33   Nicotine, when injected into an anaesthetised cat, causes an increase in systolic and diastolic blood pressure as well as an increase in heart rate.

18.34   In mice, atropine exerts a synergistic effect on the hyperkinesis induced by amphetamine.

18.35   The increase in locomotor activity in response to amphetamine is due to direct stimulation of central dopamine receptors by amphetamine.

18.36   The concentration of salicylate in saliva correlates well with plasma salicylate concentration.

18.37   The addition of adrenaline is always required in solutions of lignocaine to be used as local anaesthetics.

18.38   Wheal formation following histamine skin tests is partly due to arteriolar vasodilation.

18.39   Histamine H_2 antagonists reduce both the wheal and flare response to histamine.

18.40   Nicotine from inhaled cigarette smoke causes direct coronary vasoconstriction.

18.41   Plasma levels of lead can be determined more accurately in a carbon rod atomiser than in flame burner atomiser.

18.42   Blood lead concentrations are an accurate indicator of the total body lead burden.

18.43   β-Adrenoceptor agonists are the drugs of first choice for patients with episodic asthma.

18.44   The efficacy of frusemide as a diuretic is greater than that of chlorothiazide and amiloride.

18.45   A protein-bound drug and its unbound form can be separated by dialysis.

18.46   The concentration of acetylcholine, in a sample which is incubated *in vitro* with serum cholinesterase, decreases exponentially with time.

18.47   The rate of diffusion of a drug across a semipermeable membrane is reduced when plasma protein binding reduces the free drug concentration.

18.48   In Scatchard analysis, both total and nonsaturable binding should be determined at each radioligand concentration used in the assay.

18.49   Drugs that have affinity for receptors in binding assays may be agonists or antagonists.

CORRECT OPTION

18.50   How many milligrams of drug are there in 2 ml of 0.5% w/v solution?
   A.   1
   B.   10
   C.   100
   D.   1,000
   E.   10,000.

18.51   Dose-response curves for graded pharmacological effects are best plotted on graphs with the ordinate (vertical axis) and abscissa (horizontal axis) respectively:
    A.   both logarithmic scale
    B.   both linear scale
    C.   linear/log scale
    D.   log/linear scale
    E.   none of the above.

18.52   The modal value of a frequency distribution may be defined as its:
    A.   arithmetic average
    B.   modal item
    C.   most commonly occurring value
    D.   geometric mean
    E.   harmonic mean.

18.53   Non-parametric statistical tests:
    A.   require that the data being analysed obey a normal distribution
    B.   require that both population and sample obey a normal distribution
    C.   require only that the population conforms to a normal distribution
    D.   are independent of distribution of the data
    E.   are only used where Student's t-test fails to reject the null hypothesis.

18.54   The standard error of the mean of a series of observations:
    A.   is a measure of the scatter of the individual figures
    B.   gives an estimate of the extent to which the mean will vary if the experiment is repeated a number of times
    C.   is always greater than the standard deviation
    D.   is given by the formula   standard error = standard deviation/n where n = the number of readings
    E.   is used in the non-parametric 't-test' to see if two independent groups have been drawn from the same population.

18.55   Which of the following is an advantage of analysis of variance (F-test)?
    A.   The F-test makes fewer assumptions about the data than the t-test.
    B.   The F-test will test for a difference among several groups with one application, while the t-test requires calculation for each two-group comparison.
    C.   The F-test is more powerful than the t-test for the two-group experiment.
    D.   The value calculated for F equals t in the two group experiment and so F is usually larger than t (unless t<1).
    E.   None of the above.

18.56   What volume of a 2 mg/ml solution would be required to be given to an animal weighing 20 g to achieve a dose rate of 20 mg/kg?
    A.   0.01 ml
    B.   0.02 ml
    C.   0.1 ml
    D.   0.2 ml
    E.   0.4 ml.

18.57 To obtain a final concentration of 2×10^{-6} mol/l of noradrenaline in a 15 ml organ bath, the volume of 1×10^{-4} mol/l stock solution of noradrenaline added to the bath is:
  A. 0.15 ml
  B. 0.2 ml
  C. 0.3 ml
  D. 0.33 ml
  E. 0.5 ml.

18.58 If 0.1 ml solution of 5×10^{-4} M noradrenaline is added to a 50 ml organ bath, the final concentration of noradrenaline in the bath is:
  A. 1×10^{-7} M
  B. 2.5×10^{-7} M
  C. 1×10^{-6} M
  D. 2.5×10^{-6} M
  E. 1×10^{-5} M.

18.59 Which of the following is the most concentrated solution of atropine?
  A. undiluted 100 nmol/l
  B. a 1/10 dilution of 1 μmol/l
  C. a 1/100 dilution of 1 mmol/l
  D. undiluted 10^{-7} mol/l.

18.60 When compared to the dose-response curve for acetylcholine, the dose-response curve for choline:
  A. lies to the left, indicating lower potency
  B. lies to the right, indicating lower potency
  C. lies to the left, indicating higher potency
  D. lies to the right, indicating higher potency
  E. is the same as that for acetylcholine.

18.61 If, on a log dose-response curve for acetylcholine, an EC_{50} of 5.7×10^{-8} was obtained, a choline dose-response curve on the same preparation would show:
  A. an EC_{50} of 9.3×10^{-4} M, with a change in the maximum response
  B. an EC_{50} of 3.3×10^{-10} M, with the same maximum response
  C. an EC_{50} of 9.3×10^{-4} M, with the same maximum response
  D. an EC_{50} of 5.7×10^{-8} M, with a decreased maximum response.

18.62 The dose-response curve for acetylcholine in the presence of noradrenaline is shifted to the right of the control acetylcholine curve. This is because noradrenaline:
  A. is a muscarinic agonist
  B. is a physiological antagonist of acetylcholine
  C. is a competitive antagonist of acetylcholine
  D. displaces acetylcholine from receptor sites.

18.63 Noradrenaline, when added to an isolated guinea-pig ileum, causes the response to acetylcholine to:
  A. increase, due to an additive effect
  B. decrease, due to competition for the same receptor
  C. decrease, due to a decrease in receptor sensitivity
  D. decrease, due to physiological antagonism
  E. remain unchanged.

18.64   A solution of unknown drug, when tested on the guinea-pig ileum, did not produce a contraction. It abolished the responses to acetylcholine and nicotine. The unknown solution contained:
    A.   a muscarinic agonist
    B.   a nicotinic antagonist
    C.   a nicotinic agonist
    D.   a muscarinic antagonist
    E.   a histaminic antagonist.

18.65   When an unknown drug was tested on isolated guinea-pig ileum, the following results were found:

DRUG	RESPONSE
Unknown	contraction
Unknown + Hexamethonium	contraction
Unknown + mepyramine	contraction
Unknown + atropine	no response

The unknown may be:
    A.   acetylcholine-like
    B.   histamine-like
    C.   nicotine-like
    D.   a histamine H_1 antagonist
    E.   a ganglion blocker.

18.66   Nicotine, when administered to a guinea-pig ileum:
    A.   depolarises autonomic ganglia, initiating action potentials in postganglionic fibres
    B.   directly depolarises the smooth muscle
    C.   relaxes the ileum
    D.   antagonises the actions of acetylcholine at muscarinic receptors.

18.67   The agonist activity of:
    A.   acetylcholine at nicotinic receptors can be directly antagonised by atropine
    B.   histamine at histamine receptors can be directly antagonised by pempidine
    C.   nicotine at muscarinic receptors can be directly antagonised by atropine
    D.   acetylcholine at nicotinic receptors can be directly antagonised by pempidine.

18.68   In which group of drugs do all members produce a positive inotropic effect in isolated guinea-pig atria?
    A.   adrenaline, isoprenaline, salbutamol
    B.   isoprenaline, noradrenaline, propranolol
    C.   adrenaline, ouabain, quinidine
    D.   none of the above.

18.69   Which of the following drugs produces a negative chronotropic effect in guinea-pig atria?
    A.   noradrenaline
    B.   isoprenaline
    C.   salbutamol
    D.   carbachol
    E.   none of the above.

18.70 Which of the following drug combinations in guinea-pig atria can be used to calculate a pA_2?
    A.   adrenaline and carbachol
    B.   salbutamol and carbachol
    C.   isoprenaline and carbachol
    D.   adrenaline and propranolol
    E.   ouabain and propranolol.

18.71

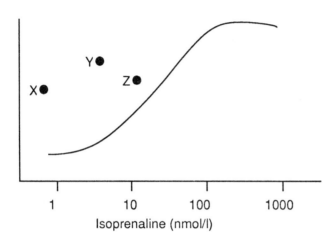

Isoprenaline (nmol/l)

A dose response curve for isoprenaline in guinea-pig isolated atria is shown above. Responses to bolus doses of three different β-adrenoceptor agonists (X, Y and Z) are also shown. The rank order of potency of X, Y and Z relative to isoprenaline is:
    A.   X > Y > Z > isoprenaline
    B.   Y > X > Z > isoprenaline
    C.   isoprenaline > Z > Y > X
    D.   isoprenaline > Y > Z > X
    E.   X > Z > Y > isoprenaline.

18.72 Which of the following inhibits contractions of the propranolol- and phentolamine-pretreated rabbit jejunum?
    A.   adrenaline
    B.   guanethidine
    C.   isoprenaline
    D.   nerve stimulation
    E.   none of the above.

18.73 Guanethidine blocks the effects of nerve stimulation in the rabbit jejunum (Finkelman) preparation by blocking:
    A.   the release of noradrenaline
    B.   uptake of noradrenaline
    C.   α-adrenoceptors
    D.   β-adrenoceptors
    E.   the synthesis of noradrenaline.

18.74

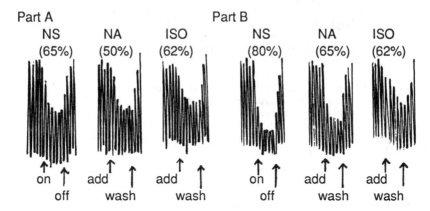

Part A   Part B
NS   NA   ISO   NS   NA   ISO
(65%)   (50%)   (62%)   (80%)   (65%)   (62%)

on ↑   add ↑   add ↑   on ↑   add ↑   add ↑
  off   wash   wash   off   wash   wash

The responses from a rabbit jejunum preparation in which the sympathetic nerve supply is intact are shown above. The % inhibition of rhythmic contractions is shown in brackets. Part A shows the control responses to nerve stimulation (NS) and doses of noradrenaline (NA) and isoprenaline (ISO). Part B shows responses to the same treatments in the presence of drug X, added 5 minutes previously.

Drug X is:
A. phentolamine
B. propranolol
C. amitriptyline
D. guanethidine
E. none of the above.

18.75   The neuromuscular block produced by suxamethonium in the rat phrenic nerve diaphragm preparation is associated with:
A. competitive antagonism
B. permanent depolarisation
C. desensitisation only
D. desensitisation followed by depolarisation
E. initial depolarisation followed by desensitisation.

18.76   The toad rectus abdominis preparation is suitable for the investigation of drugs which act on:
A. tryptaminergic receptors
B. α- and β-adrenoceptors
C. nicotinic receptors
D. cardiac muscle
E. vascular smooth muscle .

18.77   Which of the following does not have agonist properties at skeletal muscle acetylcholine receptors?
A. nicotine
B. acetylcholine
C. methacholine
D. suxamethonium
E. carbachol.

18.78   The addition of suxamethonium to the isolated toad rectus abdominis preparation produces:
   A.   no observable effect
   B.   synergism with the antagonist action of (+)-tubocurarine
   C.   competitive antagonism of the agonist action of acetylcholine
   D.   non-competitive antagonism of the agonist action of acetylcholine
   E.   a contraction, proportional to the dose administered.

18.79   High doses of acetylcholine can cause paralysis of the phrenic nerve-diaphragm preparation by:
   A.   depolarisation and desensitisation of the motor end-plate
   B.   hyperpolarisation of the motor end-plate
   C.   blockade of sodium ion transport across the muscle membrane
   D.   none of the above.

18.80   Which of the following does not produce antinociception in experimental animals after intracerebroventricular administration?
   A.   neurotensin
   B.   β-endorphin
   C.   leu-enkephalin
   D.   D-phenylalanine
   E.   corticotrophin.

18.81   Groups of mice (15 in each group) were injected with (+)-tubocurarine and then tested for their ability to maintain a grip on a rolling drum. The following results were obtained:

Group	Dose(g/kg)	Number falling off
1	1000	15
2	800	15
3	600	12
4	450	9
5	350	6
6	250	3

The ED 50 is approximately:
   A.   900 µg/kg
   B.   700 µg/kg
   C.   500 µg/kg
   D.   400 µg/kg
   E.   300 µg/kg.

18.82   A novel drug X is tested for its ability to antagonise the effects of (+)-tubocurarine in mice. Using probit analysis, the dose-response curve for (+)-tubocurarine plus drug X is shown to be shifted to the right of that of (+)-tubocurarine alone. The slopes of the dose response curves are shown to be parallel. These results indicate that:
   A.   drug X is an agonist at (+)-tubocurarine receptors
   B.   drug X is a non-competitive antagonist of (+)-tubocurarine
   C.   drug X is a competitive antagonist of (+)-tubocurarine
   D.   drug X inhibits the metabolism of (+)-tubocurarine
   E.   (+)-tubocurarine inhibits the metabolism of drug X.

18.83 The body weight of two samples of mice were compared by Student's t- test. There were 9 mice in one group and 10 in the other group. The degrees of freedom for the comparison are:
   A.   20
   B.   19
   C.   18
   D.   17
   E.   10.

18.84 The area of the brain which is thought to be the most important in amphetamine-induced locomotor activity is the:
   A.   nucleus accumbens
   B.   caudate nucleus
   C.   substantia nigra
   D.   hypothalamus
   E.   amygdala.

18.85 The locomotor stimulant effect of amphetamine:
   A.   can be blocked by reserpine
   B.   is due mainly to the release of noradrenaline
   C.   is dependent on an intact synthetic pathway for dopamine and noradrenaline
   D.   is the result of amphetamine acting on dopamine receptors
   E.   occurs *via* an indirect mechanism involving the release of granular stores of transmitter.

18.86 Which pair of drugs correctly completes the sentence below?
In an anaesthetised animal, the blood pressure and heart rate effects of .... after treatment with .... will mimic the effects of isoprenaline.
   A.   noradrenaline and phentolamine
   B.   noradrenaline and propranolol
   C.   adrenaline and phentolamine
   D.   adrenaline and propranolol
   E.   tyramine and phentolamine.

18.87 Adrenaline causes a decrease in diastolic pressure. This decrease is mainly due to:
   A.   vasoconstriction of skin and splanchnic arterioles
   B.   vasodilation of skin and splanchnic arterioles
   C.   stimulation of the vasomotor centre in the medulla
   D.   vasoconstriction of skeletal muscle arterioles
   E.   vasodilation of skeletal muscle arterioles.

18.88 An atropinised dog is given a large dose of acetylcholine which leads to an increase in blood pressure. This is because:
   A.   acetylcholine stimulates sympathetic ganglia
   B.   acetylcholine stimulates postganglionic sympathetic receptors
   C.   atropine blocks postganglionic sympathetic receptors
   D.   atropine blocks nicotinic receptors
   E.   none of the above.

18.89 An increase in heart rate is caused by all of the following drugs except:
   A.   atropine
   B.   propranolol
   C.   adrenaline
   D.   isoprenaline
   E.   phentolamine.

18.90 Physostigmine potentiates the hypotensive effect of low doses of acetylcholine in the anaesthetised dog because physostigmine:
    A.   blocks muscarinic ganglionic receptors
    B.   inhibits acetylcholinesterase
    C.   blocks the sympathomimetic actions of acetylcholine
    D.   exerts a relaxant effect on vascular smooth muscle
    E.   blocks the uptake of choline into presynaptic nerve terminals.

18.91 - 18.93

18.91   propranolol

18.92   phent lamine

18.93   pargyline

For each of the drugs listed above, indicate whether it:

    A.   blocks the depressor response to isoprenaline
    B.   increases the pressor response to tyramine
    C.   reduces the pressor response to tyramine.

18.94 Which of the following drugs is most likely to cause an increase in urinary pH?
    A.   acetazolamide
    B.   amiloride
    C.   caffeine
    D.   chlorothiazide
    E.   frusemide.

18.95 The elimination of the metabolites of a 600 mg dose of aspirin is usually completed in:
    A.   5-10 hours
    B.   10-15 hours
    C.   15-30 hours
    D.   30-40 hours.

18.96 Which of the following stimuli does not induce bronchoconstriction in subjects with asthma?
    A.   methacholine
    B.   vasoactive intestinal peptide
    C.   exercise
    D.   histamine.

18.97 Local anaesthetics:
    A.   reversibly block the generation and conduction of impulses in nerve fibres
    B.   decrease the permeability of the nerve membrane to sodium ions
    C.   are usually weak bases which exist in charged and uncharged forms at physiological pH
    D.   all of the above.

18.98 Which of the following drugs, when instilled into the eye, is most likely to cause miosis and a mild accommodation spasm?
A.   adrenaline
B.   pilocarpine
C.   tropicamide
D.   none of the above.

18.99 Which of the following graphs best describes the probability of having a crash (P) at a certain blood ethanol (BAC) level?

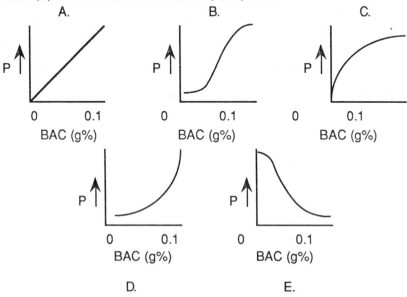

18.100 The measurements shown below were recorded before and 2 minutes after the administration of a drug.

	before drug	2 min after drug
heart rate (beats/min)	60	90
mean blood pressure (mm Hg)	87	86
plethysmograph amplitude (recorded on ear lobe)	10	13

The drug is most likely to be:
A.   nicotine (after smoking a cigarette)
B.   propranolol (i.v.)
C.   glyceryl trinitrate (sublingual).

18.101 A 60 ml post-aspirin urine sample was analysed 15 minutes after mixing with Trinder's reagent and was found to have a salicylic acid concentration of 80 mg/100 ml. The amount of salicylic acid excreted was:
A.   480 mg
B.   75 mg
C.   48 mg
D.   no valid estimate can be made due to insufficient data.

18.102 Which of the following is essential to enable comparison of the specific activities of true and pseudo-acetylcholinesterase?
    A.   use of an inhibitor of known concentration
    B.   knowledge of enzyme protein concentrations
    C.   use of a variety of substrate analogues
    D.   knowledge of the structures of the binding sites of each enzyme.

18.103 Which of the following statements is true?
    A.   Cholinesterase breaks down choline more readily than it breaks down acetylcholine.
    B.   Choline is an antagonist of acetylcholine at the muscarinic receptor.
    C.   Choline has a lower affinity than acetylcholine for the muscarinic receptor.
    D.   Choline is a physiological antagonist of acetylcholine.

18.104 Which of the following types of chemical binding is not involved in the binding of drugs to plasma protein?
    A.   ionic
    B.   hydrogen
    C.   covalent
    D.   van der Waal's forces
    E.   dipole interaction.

INCORRECT OPTION

18.105 A constant time interval between additions of an agonist drug on guinea-pig ileum is necessary because:
    A.   it reduces the number of possible sources of error
    B.   it enables reproducible contractions to be obtained
    C.   the receptors on the ileum have a refractory period of three minutes
    D.   it standardises the amount of time with which the drug is in contact with the tissue.

18.106 In the isolated guinea-pig ileum:
    A.   noradrenaline is a physiological antagonist of acetylcholine
    B.   noradrenaline causes a parallel shift in the dose-response curve to acetylcholine
    C.   atropine is a competitive antagonist of acetylcholine
    D.   maximal responses to acetylcholine are not affected by atropine
    E.   maximal responses to acetylcholine are reduced by noradrenaline.

18.107 Concerning neurotransmission in the rat phrenic nerve-diaphragm preparation:
    A.   Acetylcholine binds to nicotinic receptors.
    B.   Lignocaine blocks fast sodium channels.
    C.   Potassium chloride depolarises the muscle and nerve membranes.
    D.   Suxamethonium depolarises the nerve membranes.
    E.   Neostigmine binds to acetylcholinesterase.

18.109 Adrenaline is often given in combination with a local anaesthetic because:
  A. it localises the anaesthetic at the desired site
  B. it decreases the rate of systemic absorption of the local anaesthetic
  C. it increases the plasma protein binding of the local anaesthetic
  D. it decreases systemic toxicity.

18.109 Salicylic acid:
  A. is readily reabsorbed from kidney tubules if the urine is acid
  B. is a weak acid which exists in an ionised and non-ionised form
  C. has an increased excretion rate if ammonium chloride is co-administered
  D. is usually administered orally as acetylsalicylic acid
  E. has an irritant effect on the gastrointestinal mucosa.

18.110 Glyceryl trinitrate:
  A. has a rapid onset of action when administered sublingually
  B. is administered sublingually to avoid systemic methaemoglobinaemia
  C. produces an increase in the heart rate
  D. decreases the work load on the heart
  E. produces orthostatic hypotension.

18.111 Administration of glyceryl trinitrate results in:
  A. facial flushing
  B. reduction in post-exercise heart rate
  C. postural hypotension
  D. headache
  E. decreased cardiac work.

18.112 Nicotine:
  A. causes increased intestinal motility
  B. releases catecholamines from the adrenal medulla
  C. causes bronchoconstriction *via* a direct action on smooth muscle
  D. stimulates chemoreceptors
  E. produces tachycardia and vasoconstriction.

18.113 The effects of inhaled nicotine:
  A. include an increase in blood pressure
  B. include vasoconstriction
  C. include a decrease in heart rate
  D. on the cardiovascular system can be blocked by pentolinium
  E. are readily subject to the development of tolerance.

MCQ

18.114 Parametric statistics:
  i.   seek to determine the population mean μ and/or the the population standard deviation σ from the sample values x and s
  ii.   assume the data to be normally distributed, but tolerate some deviation from normality
  iii. require the sample to be an unbiased sample of the population
  iv.   have been largely superseded for quantitative work by non-parametric methods.

18.115 Which of the following will decrease the cardiac work load during exercise?
    i.   adrenaline
    ii.   glyceryl trinitrate
    iii.   nicotine
    iv.   propranolol
    v.   isoprenaline.

18.116 In a radioligand binding experiment, the measured total radioactivity bound comprises:
    i.   radioligand bound to specific membrane receptor sites
    ii.   radioligand bound to antagonists or agonists
    iii.   radioligand bound to non-specific sites on membranes and other insoluble components
    iv.   radioligand bound to soluble protein complexes
    v.   binding of non-radioactive ligand to specific membrane receptors.

ASSERTION / REASON

18.117 Related measures statistics (eg. the paired t-test) are frequently employed in the analysis of experimental data **BECAUSE** related measures statistics reduce subject-to-subject variation.

18.118 Non-parametric tests on the differences between sample means may be used with badly skewed data **BECAUSE** non-parametric tests make no distribution assumptions.

18.119 The pA_2 measured for atropine using acetylcholine or using choline in guinea-pig ileum are the same **BECAUSE** the maximal responses to acetylcholine and choline in the guinea-pig ileum are the same.

18.120 In the isolated rat phrenic nerve-diaphragm preparation, suxamethonium reduces the response to nerve stimulation **BECAUSE** suxamethonium is a non-depolarising neuromuscular blocker.

18.121 Neostigmine causes the toad rectus abdominis muscle to contract **BECAUSE** neostigmine is an anticholinesterase.

18.122 Pretreatment of animals with neostigmine increases the ED_{50} of (+)-tubocurarine **BECAUSE** neostigmine acts as a competitive cholinergic antagonist.

18.123 The response to tyramine after an animal has been given amitriptyline is abolished **BECAUSE** amitriptyline blocks β-adrenoceptors.

18.124 Haloperidol can inhibit amphetamine-induced locomotor stimulation **BECAUSE** haloperidol has α-adrenoceptor antagonist activity.

18.125 α-Methyl-p-tyrosine decreases brain levels of dopamine (and noradrenaline) **BECAUSE** α-methyl-p-tyrosine inhibits dopa-decarboxylase.

18.126 Amphetamine can cause locomotor excitation in mice **BECAUSE** amphetamine inhibits monoamine oxidase activity.

18.127 The wheal and flare response to intradermal histamine is reduced after combined treatment with chlorpheniramine and cimetidine **BECAUSE** cimetidine is a histamine H_2 receptor antagonist.

18.128 Aspirin displays Michaelis-Menten kinetics at higher doses (>600 mg) **BECAUSE** at doses above 600 mg, enzyme pathways for salicylic acid metabolism are saturated.

18.129 GABA modulates benzodiazepine binding **BECAUSE** benzodiazepine receptors and GABA receptors are both part of the same macromolecular complex.

18.130 A protein-bound drug will pass down a gel filtration column more slowly than an unbound drug **BECAUSE** the rate of passage through the column is proportional to molecular size.

.ANSWERS

18.1	F	18.23	F	18.45	T	18.67	D	18.89	B	18.111	B
18.2	T	18.24	T	18.46	T	18.68	A	18.90	B	18.112	C
18.3	T	18.25	F	18.47	T	18.69	D	18.91	A	18.113	C
18.4	T	18.26	F	18.48	T	18.70	D	18.92	C	18.114	A
18.5	T	18.27	F	18.49	T	18.71	A	18.93	B	18.115	C
18.6	T	18.28	F	18.50	B	18.72	E	18.94	A	18.116	B
18.7	T	18.29	F	18.51	C	18.73	A	18.95	C	18.117	A
18.8	F	18.30	F	18.52	C	18.74	C	18.96	B	18.118	A
18.9	F	18.31	T	18.53	D	18.75	E	18.97	D	18.119	B
18.10	F	18.32	T	18.54	B	18.76	D	18.98	B	18.120	C
18.11	T	18.33	T	18.55	B	18.77	C	18.99	D	18.121	D
18.12	T	18.34	F	18.56	D	18.78	D	18.100	C	18.122	C
18.13	F	18.35	F	18.57	C	18.79	A	18.101	C	18.123	C
18.14	F	18.36	T	18.58	C	18.80	E	18.102	B	18.124	B
18.15	F	18.37	F	18.59	C	18.81	D	18.103	C	18.125	C
18.16	F	18.38	T	18.60	B	18.82	C	18.104	C	18.126	B
18.17	T	18.39	F	18.61	C	18.83	D	18.105	C	18.127	B
18.18	F	18.40	F	18.62	B	18.84	A	18.106	B	18.128	C
18.19	T	18.41	T	18.63	D	18.85	C	18.107	D	18.129	A
18.20	F	18.42	F	18.64	D	18.86	C	18.108	C	18.130	D
18.21	F	18.43	T	18.65	A	18.87	E	18.109	C		
18.22	F	18.44	T	18.66	A	18.88	A	18.110	B		

Index